Loving Yourself Through Cancer

A Journey of
Hope and Inspiration

Carol Rosebrough

Editorial Credit
Suzanne Hill

Foreword Credit
Dr. Wendy L. Sparling

Reviewers
E. A. Cuticchia
Jeannetta Holliman

Photo Credit
Author's Photo: James Hill

Cover Art
Colors to Destiny by Lindsay Hill

Published by Biblio Publishing
The Educational Publisher, Inc.
1313 Chesapeake Avenue
Columbus OH 43212
www.bibliopublishing.com
www.edupublisher.com

ISBN: 978-1-62249-254-1
ISBN EBook: 978-1-62249-255-8
Library of Congress Control Number: 2015905269

Dedication

This book is dedicated to my loving and beautiful children, Suzanne Hill, John Rosebrough, Rebecca Kuper, their devoted spouses, my grandchildren Ethan Hill, Lindsay Hill, Noah Kuper and our future descendants.

My children overcame a most difficult childhood after the sudden death of their father when they were only 11, 9 and 6 years of age. Through all the trials, tribulations, traumas and heartache while we built a new life without him, we grew together and our love and support for one another have never wavered.

I think my children are amazing beings and parents. They are creating new cycles and breaking old ones to provide a better life and foundation for their children than any of us ever had. I'm honored to be their mother and witness their personal growth. I look forward to their positive influence on future generations.

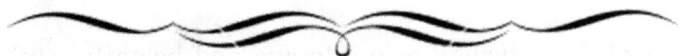

I believe that expressing

gratitude daily

multiplies the abundance

in our lives.

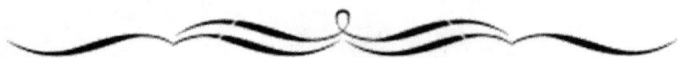

In appreciation ...

To my parents, Bessie and Lindsey Belville, who brought me into this world as their last child together at the ages of 42 and 45. Now that I know their backgrounds, I believe they did the very best they could for me and truly never meant me any harm ... especially my mother.

To John Rutledge "Jack" Rosebrough, my high school sweetheart, knight in shining armor and husband of 14 years until his sudden death at the age of 36. Jack is the first person in my life who made me feel safe. He gave me unwavering love, and we had three loving and beautiful children together.

To Elsy and John H. Rosebrough (Mimi and Pop) and Bill and Tom Rosebrough, Jack's parents and two younger brothers. This entire family unanimously adopted me as their daughter and sister from the time I was a teenager. Even though Jack has been dead for 40 years, and Mimi and Pop dead for many as well, I remain the beloved sister of Bill and Tom. Mimi served as a surrogate mother to me when I had none. She never knew I was cheated out of my own family's inheritance, but at her death, she lovingly left her meager inheritance to Bill, Tom and me ... equally. I, in turn, shared Mimi's gift equally with my children.

To Eugene A. "Gene" Cuticchia, the first and most important mentor of my life. Gene became my boss at United Cerebral Palsy of Columbus and Franklin County on the day Jack died. That very morning I received my first promotion and raise, from secretary to administrative assistant. Over the eight years we worked together, Gene was a wonderful role model. He saw me, my potential, totally supported my personal and professional growth and taught me to look within for the answers to my life. His presence was life altering for me, in a most positive way, and for that I will be eternally grateful. Because of his influence, I developed the courage, skills and heart to build the dream life I live today.

To David W. "Dave" Metz, who risked hiring me as the Division Business Manager for Times Mirror Cable Television, Inc. ... my first job in cable. That started my career which spanned 24 years, four companies, two states and helped me build the retirement plan which supports me financially today.

To James D. "Jim" Munchel, who risked retaining me as the general manager of the cable system I managed in Pennsylvania when his parent company, Susquehanna Pfaltzgraff, became the third owner. Jim had a general manager in Rhode Island, already working for him, who was expecting to replace me when her position was eliminated at the closing of the sale. Instead Jim retained me. Over the ten years we worked together, Jim's support for me was endless. My territory was quadrupled, he promoted me to the vice president level and the company recognized me with many awards, including nominating and supporting me as a participant in the industry's prestigious Betsy Magness Leadership Institute.

To Swami Shantanand "Shantji" Saraswati, a loving and devoted friend, ever since we met in Pennsylvania in 1990. Born, raised and educated in Allahabad, India he now shares his time between his Ashram on the Ganges River in Allahabad and his home and Shanti Temple in Montrose, Pennsylvania. Shantji also has a cave in India where he lived many years honing his beliefs and where he discovered his philosophy of the *Wisdom of Non Doing.* He promotes living a regulated life and living with truth on all levels in your life.

To Jeannetta Holliman, the founder of the International Women's Writing Guild regional chapter in central Ohio, and the founder and creator of the Gillie Writers Workshop. Jeannetta has given me personal support and encouragement of my writing. She used her creativity and publishing skills to take the Gillie writers on a journey ... a writing journey. And together, 15 of very diverse and ordinary senior women created and published an anthology entitled ... *Works in Process: Women Over 50 Reflecting.* This was my first experience with a formal book launch, reading and reception. It was great fun to experience this celebration with all the contributing authors. After the reading I felt like a celebrity when guests asked for my signature for their books!

To Jeanne Marlowe, the current International Women's Writing Guild regional coordinator for central Ohio. Jeanne has always offered me support, encouraged my writing and introduced me to Jeannetta.

To the doctors who have helped me navigate the healing of my body to excellent health: Dr. Wendy Sparling, my personal physician, who manages my health care on a regular basis and refers me to specialists; Dr. Jason Barfield, my neurologist, who manages my post stroke care; Dr.

Ramona Nixon, my dermatologist; Dr. George Calloway, Jr., the ophthalmologist who referred me to Dr. Gallo; Dr. Samuel Gallo, an eye and facial plastic surgeon, who biopsied and diagnosed my lymphoma cancer; Dr. Mark Davanzo, a general surgeon, who surgically implanted my port needed for chemotherapy infusions; Dr. Taral Patel, my oncology specialist, and all the other medical and administrative staff at The Mark H. Zangmeister Center, who have and continue to expertly guide me through the maze of chemotherapy and healing. My cancer treatment could have been a scary and lonely process, but instead I have always felt welcome, cared about and safe working with everyone at Zangmeister.

To every person and organization dedicated to curing and eliminating cancer, and those working every day to heal patients with cancer. Critical cancer research leads to technological and medical improvements in diagnosis and treatment. Continuous improvement in treatment results in more people not only surviving a cancer diagnosis and treatment, but going on to live a full and healthy life.

Foreword

"You have cancer." Words no one wants to hear. Carol Rosebrough's book, *Loving Yourself Through Cancer,* takes us through her journey of hearing and responding to this diagnosis. More specifically, DECIDING how to respond to the cancer diagnosis. Even more importantly, it helps us understand some truths that can help us live more fulfilled, healthier, happier, and empowered lives. These lessons are important whether or not we have had a diagnosis of cancer:

--"I forgive you." When sincere, these words are very powerful. Carol shows that when we are able to let go of things that hurt us (the process of forgiving), we are then free to heal and grow. She reminds us that forgiving does not mean we condone or forget the wrong that was done; however, it does mean that the wrong we forgive no longer has any power over us, our attitude, decisions, or responses. We become free to realize that we alone are fully responsible and can take charge of our decisions, time, health, spiritual well-being, finances, and happiness. She also reminds us that sometimes we need to forgive ourselves for things that we've done or decisions we've made in the past.

--"I'm grateful." Our attitude is so important when it comes to being as healthy as we can. Throughout this book, Carol shows us that we can find the positive lessons and learn when life throws things at us that we sometimes only want to react to as negative experiences. Even a journey through cancer treatment can make us stronger, happier, more fulfilled people. We learn that we have a lot for which to be grateful. God does send us many blessings but sometimes we miss feeling blessed due to our attitude. We fail to reap the benefits because we only perceive the event (diagnosis, accident, etc) as negative and react to it as such.

--Carol proves to us that we can change our health, habits, circumstances, etc at any age. We cannot use the excuse of "it is too late" to change for the better. As a physician, I especially like Carol's healthy approach to weight management ... not a "diet" but a "permanent lifestyle change." Almost anyone can be very successful with this approach. I hope perhaps a cookbook or some recipes online are in her future! This book helps us to understand that our relationship with our bodies is "until death do us part" and inspires us to take better care of the earthly shell which we are dependent on until death.

This book is inspiring in so many ways. It can help us face adversities in a positive, grateful, healthy way. We learn to focus on what we can do to help ourselves versus being victims of our circumstances. I wish that I could have read this book before I had to deal with my own cancer diagnosis and many other "curveballs" that life has thrown. It offers valuable tools for adults of all ages to use to come out of life's challenges as more fulfilled, more empowered, happier, and healthier people.

Dr. Wendy L. Miller-Sparling
Sunbury Square Family Medicine

Introduction

There is no such thing as a "one size fits all" response to a cancer diagnosis. Quite the opposite in fact. Each person receiving a diagnosis of cancer is different; their life experiences are different, their particular cancer is different, the condition of their body is different, the stage of their cancer is different, their treatment is different and their emotional and physical response to the cancer and treatment will be different.

Cancer is quite mysterious actually. There is no warning for it and there is no blanket vaccine against it. And cancer does not discriminate. It crosses all boundaries of race, gender, age and socio-economic status.

Cancer research has come a long way. With the advances continually made in research, odds are improved every day for people to heal their specific cancer and never have it return. Perhaps one day research will be able to eliminate cancer completely, or at least eliminate any deaths occurring as a result of it.

This book, *Loving Yourself Through Cancer*, is an outgrowth of my diagnosis of an incurable, slow growing lymphoma cancer and my healing process. It has been a transformational experience for me to write this book concurrently as I've been going through my own chemotherapy treatment.

Because I believe there are no accidents and there is a lesson to be learned from every event that happens, I approached my cancer diagnosis from the beginning looking for whatever lessons there might be for me. I was also able to incorporate and use personal growth and healing tools that I have developed over the past decades to help and guide me.

All my healing tools and the lessons I learned while going through the cancer diagnosis and chemotherapy treatment process are included in this book. One lesson, previously learned, became solidified for me and another lesson has catapulted me to an entirely new level of existence.

Writing is therapy for me. Definitely writing about my diagnosis and treatment of cancer has been healing for me personally. Accepting, appreciating, loving and taking care of my body is my lesson that became solidified during this process. My surprise lesson was that writing this book evolved into a "coming out" for me in sharing the shame and secrets of my past.

My hope now is that my story, truthfully shared in this book, will inspire others to accept, appreciate, love and take care of their bodies as well as to share their stories. It is only what is hidden that can keep us prisoners. A diagnosis of cancer is a call to heal oneself. Look within. Forgive. Heal. Grow. Become your very best self and live the life of your dreams.

Carol Rosebrough

Contents

Exhibits

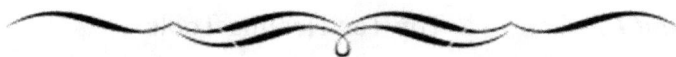

I believe just one person,

acting with kindness and love,

can shift the world.

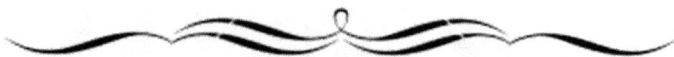

Chapter 1

What do you mean I have cancer?

I'm sitting in a black leather examining chair ready for an eye exam. It is quite similar to Dr. Calloway's office, the ophthalmologist who referred me to this specialist in eye and facial plastic surgery. I've never met with a plastic surgeon before, and I wonder what it will be like ... and more importantly what I'll find out about this lump under my left lower eyelid.

The door opens, and Dr. Gallo enters the room with an assistant. His smile is so big and energetic, it's contagious. It feels good to be here.

"Well, Carol, what brings you here to see us today?" he asks me.

"I have a lump under my left eyelid that I've had for quite a while. Dr. Sparling, my personal physician, at first thought it was a clogged duct. But when I started experiencing some double vision she referred me to Dr. Calloway, an ophthalmologist.

When he examined me he said he thought it was a fatty deposit, but he could also see that my left eye was tilting upward. He thought the lump was probably causing my vision problems. He said that my eyes were actually healthy,

1

and since his specialty was inside the eye, I needed to see someone with a specialty for outside the eye. So, that's the long version of why I'm here to see you today. Dr. Calloway referred me to you."

Dr. Gallo moves closer to me, starts feeling the lump, comparing my left lower eyelid area to my right, moves back, chats with his assistant a moment and then returns to me. "Well, I don't know what it is, but it isn't a fatty deposit. It mimics one, and is probably benign, but it should be removed, if possible, or at least I need to get a slice for a biopsy. If you're agreeable, I would like to schedule you for surgery right away to find out what this is."

"Of course, I want to know, too," I reply.

Dr. Gallo did say he thought it was benign, right? I can't have cancer. I've spent decades cleaning up and healing my past, living a spiritual life, being responsible, harming no one, and living with love, kindness and compassion for others. This will be benign for sure.

Surgery is on an outpatient basis. While I'm still in the recovery area, the normally energetic and smiling Dr. Gallo approaches me a little somberly. "I couldn't remove the lump. It was too close to the eye to remove without damaging critical eye muscles, but I did get a slice for a biopsy. It looks funny though. I think it's some low level form of lymphoma that can probably be treated with a few radiation treatments. We'll know for sure when the biopsy results are completed."

My first shock wave. No results for sure, but Dr. Gallo is preparing me to hear a diagnosis of cancer. Again, I'm in disbelief. Surely he is wrong and the diagnosis will come back as benign. Of course I'm in denial of what is happening to me.

Monica, the director of nursing, who has been caring for me pre and post op knows I want to know the results as quickly as possible, and she even offers to call me with the results over the weekend, if they are available. Unfortunately they aren't and I have to wait several days for her personal phone call to me with the results.

I'm expecting a benign diagnosis, so her call dashes my spirits. "Hello Carol, Dr. Gallo's visual diagnosis during surgery was correct. I wish it were wrong, but he's gifted in this way and usually right. The biopsy confirms the lump in your left orbit is B Cell Lymphoma. Your follow up visit with the doctor is tomorrow, and he can talk to you then about your options and next steps." I can feel Monica's concern and compassion for me as she continues ... "I'm sorry. You take care and we'll see you tomorrow."

My second shock wave. I do have cancer! But why? What does this mean? What am I supposed to learn from this? I'm still having trouble comprehending this is even a possibility of happening to me, let alone it is actually happening to me!

Unfortunately I'm not finished with the layers of shock I will experience as I enter this world of cancer, beginning with my follow up visit with Dr. Gallo to hear his recommendations.

Here I am again, in the same room and chair as in my first visit. But I'm no longer the naive person with no cancer. *At least it's only in my eye, right? And a few treatments of radiation will take it away, right?*

Then Dr. Gallo enters the room, back to his normal energetic and smiling self. He goes over the diagnosis again, reaffirming that a few treatments of radiation should clear it up. He also advises me that I can go to Ohio State or The Zangmeister Center for treatment and that I will receive the same level of care at either place. It's just a matter of convenience and where I would prefer to go for treatment.

Then comes the next shock, when he says "They'll want to do a full body scan to find out if this is anywhere else in your body."

That thought never occurred to me. Now I don't have just a cancer lump contained in my left eye orbit that can be treated with a few treatments of radiation, it could be anywhere throughout my body! I have had this lump a really long time. Maybe it has already spread everywhere throughout my body. *What would that mean for treatment? Chemotherapy? I have heard nothing but horror stories about what people experience in chemotherapy. Again, what on earth does all this mean to me? How in the world do I process it?*

My denial shifts into some fear ... fear of the unknown and what I am about to experience. I have no frame of reference to know what to expect. I haven't even had the experience of a close friend going through cancer to be able to grasp it.

What I do have, however, is an unwavering belief that anything that happens always works for my highest good, a belief that I know will sustain me throughout this experience. I'm always looking for the silver lining. Always looking for what I need to learn. Always looking for the message or the lesson.

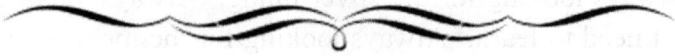

I believe there are no accidents,

only lessons to learn.

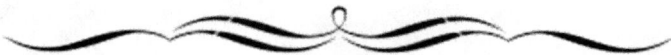

Chapter 2

Getting the Details

During my follow up visit with Dr. Sparling, I choose to use The Mark H. Zangmeister Center on the east side of Columbus for treatment and she makes the arrangements for my first appointment with them.

This is all new to me. I have never heard of this center before, but it is much more convenient for me to use for ongoing treatments. I do check out their website and find good reviews, but I come to my first visit with a great deal of apprehension. The large three story brick building with enormous windows and a large canopy at the entrance make it look more like a hotel, very pleasant, very inviting.

Registration is also pleasant and the building has a nice, light even peaceful feeling inside. So far so good. Lab work is next and then I meet with Dr. Patel, who will be my oncology specialist. He's also very nice and begins by asking what brings me to The Zangmeister Center.

I explain the litany to him with the final step being the biopsy, the diagnosis of cancer, and my decision to use Zangmeister for my treatment.

Dr. Patel then scoots on his roller chair closer to me holding some test results and a yellow legal pad. "Carol, have you seen your actual test results?"

"No," I reply, "but I would love to see them."

He shows the results to me and explains them. "Your test results confirm your lump is B Cell Lymphoma Non Hodgkins cancer with 89% CD20s concentration on the cells." He draws a picture for me on his yellow pad and the cell looks like a satellite loaded with antenna all over it. He then proceeds to tell me that the recommended treatment is chemotherapy.

And then I blurt out ... "But the doctor who performed my biopsy thought just a few treatments of radiation would be sufficient to clear this up! Is that not really possible now?"

"No, Carol. With the size and position of this cancer under your eye, I don't recommend radiation as it could cause the loss of your eyesight. The cancer is treatable with chemotherapy, but this particular type of cancer is only treatable, it's not curable."

"So, what does that mean exactly?"

"It means we can make this cancer go away now, but it could come back in the future, even as long as ten years from now."

My heart sinks and my legs go numb. Now, not only do I have cancer, I'll have to live with that it could come back sometime in the future. I think my entire body has gone into shock with the news. I can't comprehend yet that my particular type of cancer is incurable. What I focus on instead is that it's treatable.

Dr. Patel begins telling me about my recommended treatment while he is writing it down for me on his yellow pad. "We'll use R CVP chemo treatment, which stands for Rituximab, Cyclophosphamide, Vincristine, and Prednisone. The Rituximab attaches to the CD20s and specifically works on that part of the cell. The Cyclophosphamide and Vincristine are the chemo drugs, and Prednisone is a steroid, which helps curb some of the side effects of the chemo treatment. You'll need approximately 6 to 8 treatments which will last 18 to 24 weeks.

But first we'll need to do some tests to see if this is anywhere else in your body. We will schedule you for two different appointments for the tests. First we'll do PET (Positron Emission Tomography) scans for your brain and your body. Then on the second visit we'll do a bone marrow and a bone biopsy."

I'm feeling afraid and it must show on my face because Dr. Patel asks me if I want to change my mind about proceeding with the treatment, but I reply "No, I want to do this. It's just a lot for me to take in today."

"How are your veins?" he asks me.

"Oh, my veins are terrible. Everyone has trouble taking blood as the veins are so small and so deep plus they seem to run away when a needle approaches!"

Dr. Patel looks at my right arm to check out what I have just said and he agrees. "You'll need a port placement. Do you have a surgeon?"

"I have an orthopedic surgeon."

"No, you'll need a general surgeon. I'll refer you to one to get the port installed prior to beginning your therapy. Your veins will never hold up in chemotherapy treatment without it. They'll schedule you for that."

As we finish our time together, Dr. Patel tears off the sheet from his yellow pad for me to take with me. I'm grateful for something to review later, as my head is virtually swimming with all the details. He then walks with me to the area where I'll be scheduled for all the upcoming appointments.

This is Friday, the first of August. I've only known I have cancer since July 22nd. It has all moved very quickly since Dr. Sparling referred me to Dr. Calloway in June. I'm grateful to all these doctors, who did not dismiss me, but kept sending me on until I had an answer about what was happening in my eye.

I'm especially grateful to Dr. Calloway who referred me to Dr. Gallo, who actually diagnosed the cancer. I think they saved my life as there was no indication I was ill in any other way. I was feeling very healthy and strong from eating well and exercising daily for the past year, all my blood work was right in the optimal level of normal in every category and my blood pressure completely normal without taking any blood pressure medication. There wasn't one bit of evidence that anything was wrong anywhere in my body, other than this lump under my left lower eyelid.

So now I begin the process of finding out how much cancer I have and where it is in my body. Before leaving the registration area on this first visit with Dr. Patel, I'm scheduled on Tuesday the 5th of August for the brain and body scans, and on Thursday the 7th for the bone marrow and bone biopsies. My port placement surgery in the hospital is scheduled on Tuesday, August 12 with Dr. Davanzo. And my first chemo treatment is scheduled for August 18th. It seems that everything is operating at lightning speed ever since my diagnosis. I suppose it's a good thing not to waste any time getting started with treatment.

When I get to my car, I call my daughter Suzanne to give her the news of what I've just heard from the doctor and what I'm about to begin.

Suzanne is terrified of the news and yells at me, "Mom, you need to get a second opinion! You were only supposed to need radiation for three or four weeks and now you are scheduled for chemotherapy for six months! This can't be right."

Suzanne never yells at me and she usually never gives me unsolicited advice. But her fear, coming out in anger, puts me into further shock. At first I'm stunned and can't even speak.

Eventually the words come, "Suzanne, I like this place and I like this doctor." I explain to her what the doctor said about possibly losing my eyesight from the radiation and that even though it's not what I was expecting, I'm comfortable with this treatment plan. She calms down a bit, but she's obviously not okay about all of it.

I came to this appointment alone. I am absolutely on overload from all the information I've just heard. I was already in fear just having cancer under my left eye. Today I find out it could come back in the future, even if they heal it now; my tests to find out where else it is will include bone and bone marrow biopsies; my cancer treatment will be chemotherapy lasting several months and I will need surgery before I even start chemotherapy!

There is no way I can process everything before I start the drive home. My mind is racing and my body feels numb. I'm scared about even trying to drive in this condition, so I drive very, very slowly knowing that my reflexes are not normal right now. I do my best to stay as far away as possible from the other cars on the highway so that I can get home safely.

Chapter 3

Preparing for Chemotherapy

Now that I know for sure I'll be going through chemotherapy instead of radiation, I can't wait to see what I can find on the Internet about it.

The first thing I learn is that the treatment prescribed by Dr. Patel at Zangmeister is exactly what I find on the Internet as the best treatment for the type cancer I have. That actually helps me relax. But then I read further about side effects and the dangers of infection.

Even though my cancer is incurable, I've been told by the doctors it's considered very treatable so I don't think I'm in any danger of dying from the cancer. And I've never heard of anyone dying from chemotherapy itself. However, what I have heard is that people are very vulnerable to infection while going through chemotherapy due to a compromised immune system, a side effect from the treatment. And at 74 years of age, I think it's possible I could die if I get a serious infection during chemotherapy.

I don't want to die. I know that. More than that, I want to be healthy and fit so that I can really enjoy my life to the fullest. I have a lot to live for and enjoy; children, grandchildren, my own life and I have lots I still want to accomplish. However, my age is definitely a factor making me more vulnerable to infection while going through chemotherapy. The Internet has many different lists with ways to prevent infection. I realize it will take some time to absorb all the information and know which ones are important for me to use.

But, I realize there is a bigger problem. My adult son John lives with me now and he's very prone to getting sick, and often. On the one hand I like the idea he is living with me. I think it could be good if he helped me get through cancer treatment, but on the other, can I risk him infecting me with a cold which could turn into pneumonia?

This is very tricky. John and I get along very well now, but we didn't when he was younger. I don't want to hurt him, but perhaps him living with me while I'm in chemotherapy isn't a good idea. I wonder if he will move back in with Amber, his girlfriend. He has tried living with her before, only to end up moving back in with me. I'll ask him, but I'm not sure how he'll feel about living with her again.

I don't look forward to this conversation as I don't want to cause any damage to him and our relationship. I meditate before talking to him to make sure I'm centered and able to speak with him in love.

When we get together I tell him I have something I want to talk to him about. "John, I'm worried about going through chemotherapy. I'm not worried about the cancer, and I'm not worried about the chemotherapy, but I'm terrified about the possibility of getting an infection, which could kill me. Since you get sick often, I think it would be a good idea if you moved out ... just while I am receiving chemotherapy. If

Amber would let you move in with her, that would work great. It's not that I don't want you here, I just don't want to risk getting an infection while going through treatment."

"Mom, I definitely don't want to take you out with a cold. I know Amber would love for me to move back in, so maybe that's what I should do. I just need to know ... will you save my room for me and let me move back in for sure when this is all over?"

"I promise, John. I'll save your room for you and you'll be welcome to move back in just as soon as I'm healthy enough and not in danger. Your moving out is only a means to protect me from getting an infection. It's not because I don't want you to live with me. Unfortunately there is no guarantee that I still won't get an infection, but living alone will certainly make it easier to prevent one."

"Okay, Mom. If this will help you, I'll talk to Amber. I'm sure she'll love me moving back in, and for her the sooner the better."

"Thanks, John, I really appreciate your willingness to do this for me."

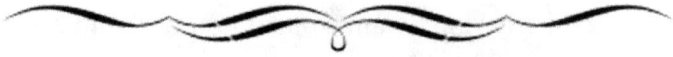

I believe that something good emerges

from every event, regardless of how it

appears at the moment.

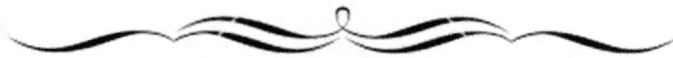

Chapter 4

Steps to Prevent Infection

John moving in with Amber definitely removes one huge potential infection risk for me. I can close off the upstairs, which is where he lives when with me. However, after my research on the Internet, I realize there are many more things I need to do if I am serious about protecting myself from infection.

Washing my hands consistently seems to be the main priority. I already have antibiotic liquid hand soap dispensers in both downstairs bathrooms and the kitchen, but I haven't always been consistent about washing my hands. Now I have no choice. I have no margin of error and must do everything I can to protect myself. I also decide to place a roll of paper towels in each bathroom and in the kitchen so that I can dry my hands, throw away the paper towel and stay more sanitary than reusing a cloth hand towel every time I wash my hands.

I place a can of sanitizing wipes in all the same locations. They're extremely handy to quickly clean the light switches, door knobs, sink handles, soap dispenser pumps, toilet handles and toilet seats.

For over twenty five years I've had someone else clean my house every other week. But this past January, I decided to start doing that for myself. Although I wonder if that's still the best plan, I realize I don't want someone else coming into the house risking an infection. I know I'm most vulnerable to an infection right after treatment, so before my first chemo treatment I thoroughly sanitize both bathrooms, and I change my bed linens.

Since I'm living alone, sharing towels is not a problem, but normally I use the same towel and wash cloth more than once. I decide not to reuse them at all. I shower every day, and I make a plan. A load of laundry every day can include my clothes from the day before, the bath towel and wash cloth and my pajamas from the night before. If I can keep up with it every day, it won't be a burden.

Face masks and plastic gloves are the next items to add. I think these are needed when I go out in public, or when I'm vacuuming or dusting in the house. My vacuum has the canister that has to be emptied and dust scatters easily. A mask will help me prevent inhaling the dirt I have just swept up or dusted.

I also decide not to attend any writing groups, nor any other group, while going through chemotherapy. I'm not willing to risk the possibility of being exposed to someone who might be sick. But I need to shop for groceries and may need to be in other places where I will not be able to control who is there. I will need the face mask and gloves for those times.

I have significant sleep apnea and it is critical that I use the CPAP (Continuous Positive Airway Pressure) equipment every night. I already change my face liner every day, but not always the mask. I decide to wash and change my mask every day and at least once a week to wash and sanitize all the other parts.

The CPAP hose, filter, humidifier, lid and lid liner can all be washed with dish detergent. I separate the two parts of the machine and use sanitizing wipes to clean the air holes and the interior and exterior of the machine. Since I'm breathing air from this machine and these attachments all night long, every night, I think I can't be too careful about avoiding infection from any part of it. The other preventions I start are to hang up the hose every morning plus empty the humidifier so they both have a chance to dry out during the day before reusing that night.

The other important item is my nutrition and having food ready before I begin chemotherapy. I wash all my fruit and vegetables before eating or cutting. I even wash the fruit with a rind or skin that isn't eaten (lemons, limes, oranges, melons) because without washing it first, the bacteria on the skin can transfer from the knife to the fruit inside. With all my vegetables clean and ready, I make an enormous pot of lentil and vegetable soup, freezing in two cup portions to have available over the next few weeks. I have other fresh vegetables and fruit ready as well. I've done everything I can think of to protect myself from infection and to have nutritional food prepared in advance. I think I'm ready to begin chemotherapy.

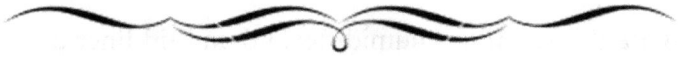

I have come to learn that my inner guidance is always right.

The more I trust and follow it, I am led to the best possible outcome in any situation.

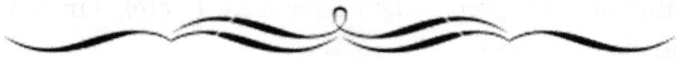

Chapter 5

Getting Started

Last Friday I saw Dr. Patel for the first time. Now it is Tuesday, 7:15 AM and I'm back at Zangmeister for the brain and body scans. A six-hour fasting was required before the tests, but that is easy for me since I don't ever eat in the evenings anymore.

But I'm nervous about what the test results will reveal about my cancer. Do I have it throughout my body? I have been disassociated from my body most of my life and have never felt for lumps before. I start feeling my neck, arms and my legs and I find lumps. *Lots* of small lumps, especially in my arms and legs. My only conclusion is that the cancer has already spread throughout my body. I find a lump by my right knee and Dr. Patel schedules extra time for that part of my body to be tested, too.

I'm slightly claustrophobic, so having three scans, two for the brain and one for the body, increases my anxiety. I use meditation in this situation to remove myself from the machine so that I can tolerate the close confinement and inability to move for a long period of time. I concentrate on my breath and try to keep myself centered. It works. The time passes more quickly than I imagine possible. Okay. Step one completed.

On Thursday I return to Zangmeister for the bone marrow and bone biopsies. I'm more than nervous about these tests, I am terrified. It's really hard to calm myself down. I'm blessed with the workers at Zangmeister as they're not only very competent in their medical skills, they are nice people and do their best to put me at ease.

Two people are with me for these biopsies. My hip area is numbed with a shot and I'm told the numbing will work for the bone marrow extraction, but the bone will not be numb. I'm totally awake for the procedure. The bone marrow biopsy is relatively simple, painless and doesn't take long. The nurses engage me in conversation about my family as a distraction and it helps.

The bone biopsy is a little different and I'm expecting the worst. The nurse has me on my side and then begins rocking my hip back and forth, presumably loosening a piece of the bone from the same area the bone marrow was extracted. Mostly I feel pressure rather than pain, and it's over pretty quickly. It is far easier than I expected. I think the person doing the extraction must be superb in her skill level.

Now that the tests are over, I sit up and prepare to leave. But then the nurse who extracted the bone marrow asks if I would like to see it.

"I would love to see it!"

She picks up two vials, one containing my bone marrow and one the bone chip. I fully expected bone marrow to be a solid mass, but it isn't at all. It's a liquid, a dark red liquid, and she moves the vial back and forth for me to see the consistency. It's amazing. It looks more like blood. The piece of bone that was extracted is floating in some form of liquid as well. This is quite an education for me and I love it. Now I'll be able to visualize my bone marrow!

And then I ask them, "So where do you send these for the biopsy?"

"There is only one place, a company in California. It's the only company that can actually do these biopsies."

No wonder scheduling of everything was so tricky. There needed to be enough time to get these results back before I had the follow up meeting with the doctor and my first chemotherapy treatment. As we finish up, the nurses box up my bone marrow and bone sample for the shipment. Very efficient.

On Tuesday I have my surgical appointment to have the port placement installed. This part didn't sound complicated to me when I was told about it originally, but in the meeting with Dr. Davanzo, the surgeon, I realize it is complicated.

He explains the procedure will be done at the hospital on an outpatient basis, and I will not be fully sedated. I will only have some form of a twilight solution. He has a sample device of what he will use for me, and demonstrates how it works.

It's a small round hard plastic device attached to a long thin soft plastic tubing. The round device is the actual port to be used for the chemotherapy drugs infusion, and it will be surgically implanted under the skin in my chest. The attached tubing will also be placed under the skin wrapping around to be inserted into a vein in my neck.

I'm concerned about where in my neck this is to be placed as I don't want it in the carotid artery. After having a warning stroke (TIA Transient Ischemic Attack) last year and knowing I already have some plaque blockage in my carotid arteries, I certainly don't want something else in there that will possibly create more problems. Dr. Davanzo assures me it will not be placed in my carotid artery, and I am relieved.

The port serves as the entry point for the IV chemo drug infusions, and then the drugs travel through the tubing into the vein in the right side of my neck. With this system, they are able to enter my body effortlessly. And because I receive several different drugs for each treatment, this system makes changes between one drug and the next extremely simple. The nurses just stop the flow of one drug entering the IV, disconnect it, and then start the next one. I can even be sleeping when they make the change. It's amazing there is such a reliable system for this process without needing to use the veins in my arms.

It takes me a few days to recover from this surgery. I find I need to sit up while sleeping and bending over is difficult. Otherwise I have a pounding sensation of blood rushing to the port site, and pain not only in the port site but my neck as well. I'm grateful I decided in advance to board my dog Buddy for the surgery and recovery process. I would never have been able to bend over getting him ready to go in and out, preparing his food, or even taking him for his daily walks during this time.

Monday is my next appointment with Dr. Patel and also my first chemo treatment. I've had all the tests now, and I'll hear the results. I'm ready to begin chemotherapy, but I've worked myself into quite a state worrying about how much cancer is in my body.

My daughter Suzanne has driven me to this appointment and we hear the news together. Dr. Patel begins, "Carol, we have all the test results and I'm pleased to tell you there is no cancer in your body anywhere, except under your left eye." We are both elated, relieved and grateful with this news.

Then I ask him, "Well, what about the lumps I felt on my arms and legs? Are they just fatty deposits then?"

He smiles, "Yes, that is what they are. They're not cancer." He pauses for a moment to let me absorb this wonderful news before continuing, "You'll be treated with six rounds of chemotherapy at 21 day intervals. You'll be monitored during each one to see how you are tolerating the treatment. The speed of the infusion drugs entering your body will increase as you are able to tolerate it. The Rituximab will take the longest, several hours in fact. You'll be here most of the day for treatment. And then 24 hours after your chemo treatment you'll come back for a Neulasta shot. It's a booster shot to activate building more white blood cells in your bone marrow to help offset what you lose from the chemo treatment."

I like this news. With all my reading on the Internet about my type of cancer, treatments and side effects, I never saw anything about getting a white blood cell booster shot. It reassures me I'm getting the best possible treatment, and I'm glad I'm coming here.

I have a question that has been on my mind ever since I got the diagnosis, "Dr. Patel, now that I know the only cancer I have is under my left eye, I think I know how I got it. Sometime after I retired, a few years ago, I got an infection on my eyelid in the very spot where I have cancer now. It was from using old mascara and it slipped and I must have gotten something on my lid or in my eye. It was only treated with eye wash at the time. Could this be the source with abnormal cells forming around the foreign object and infected area?"

"No, I think it's more likely you had the cancer first and that caused the infection. This is a very slow growing cancer so it would have taken a long time to build to this point."

I'm a little worried that I might still have something in my eye from that slip with the mascara, so I ask Dr. Patel, "When you do the next PET scan will you be able to see if there is still a speck of mascara under my eyelid?"

"No, Carol. We won't be able to detect such a speck, but I wouldn't worry about that. The body is a wonderful cleaning machine and it would have already removed the speck out of your body."

If I don't have cancer throughout my body then perhaps the treatment will not be as severe as I've been expecting. I guess I'll find out today since I'm receiving my first chemotherapy treatment. Suzanne and I leave the first floor and go to the second floor for me to register for the chemo infusion.

Suzanne is only allowed to spend a few minutes with me off and on in the chemo infusion area during the day, but it doesn't matter. She wants to know how I'm progressing. She either waits in the car, or in the waiting area, and periodically comes to check on me to see if there is anything I need. I try to convince her to leave and come back at the end of the day, but she stays. In the end, I'm grateful. Her presence and checking on me throughout the day is more comforting than I imagine possible.

The chemo infusion area is quite nice. Large leather lounge chairs are placed throughout the area in small clusters. I'm lucky. My seat today is facing a window wall and I have a view of a large tree line outside. It's quiet and I like not facing anyone else and having the view. I'm very grateful now that I have the port in my chest for the infusion. I'm not really over the surgery for the port placement yet, and still have a bandage over the incision, but that's okay. I have Lidocaine cream to numb the port area before treatment.

The nurse has a kit she uses that contains what she needs for me, plus everything for herself as well. She even has a manual that gives me highlights about what I can expect from Zangmeister, my treatment and possible side effects. She goes through each section with me, and then it's mine to take home as a reference.

Knowing that I would be here for treatment for several hours, I brought a container of raspberry lemonade Crystal

Light and some nutritious food to have during the day. Unfortunately I only brought one drink container on this first visit and it doesn't last all day. The center offers coffee, tea and juice for patients, and I take an apple juice late in the day. It tastes so sweet to me though I can hardly drink it. I decide I'll bring two or three containers of my favorite raspberry lemonade on my next visit.

The Rituximab takes about four hours to enter my body on this first visit. The other drugs all take much less time. I'm quite cold during the infusion, either from the temperature in the room or the emotional shock I'm in, or both. The nurse ends up giving me three warm blankets before I finally stop shivering. The fluorescent overhead lighting also hurts my eyes, and I decide to bring something on the next visit to cover them.

I'm exhausted when the treatment is over. My body definitely is in shock now and I feel shaky in general. I steady myself by holding onto my daughter's arm as we walk out of the chemo infusion area. I'm so grateful that she is with me and I don't have to drive myself home.

We don't leave the center until about 5PM. My chemotherapy treatment has lasted the entire day. We encounter all the rush hour traffic on the highway. It takes longer than normal to get home, but I have the seat back, my eyes closed and try to relax during the drive. Suzanne comes inside my home with me to make sure I get settled before she leaves. Fortunately I have everything ready for myself. I walked Buddy this morning, so all I need to do is let him outside for a few moments, then get undressed and climb into my clean bed for the night.

My first treatment is over. I wonder what kind of reaction I'll have.

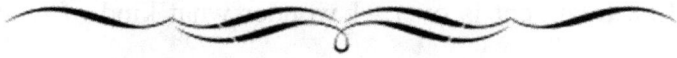

I believe every crisis can

lead us to create a new way of being.

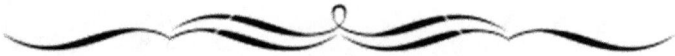

Chapter 6

Initial Side Effects

The first few days following treatment I have multiple side effects. My fear increases as they get worse with each passing day. The first one comes from the Prednisone, which is to help curb side effects from the chemo drugs. I haven't had any caffeine to drink for a year, so this steroid hits my body with full force. My mind and body are racing, I can't stop moving and I lie awake all night with thoughts racing through my mind.

I'm only on a five day dose of Prednisone following treatment and was told to take it early in the morning or it could prevent me from sleeping. Evidently I didn't take it early enough today, so I set the alarm for tomorrow morning at 5 AM. I needn't have bothered. My mind doesn't settle down during the night and I don't think I sleep at all. I take the prescribed four pills shortly after I get up, but the earlier hour doesn't seem to make any difference.

I'm worried about being so hyper. On the one hand it can be good as I'll definitely get a lot done, but I wonder what will happen when I stop taking the Prednisone?

I'm also nauseous. I know I tend to get nauseous easily, and Dr. Patel prescribed an anti nausea medication for me that has worked well for me in the past. But as I'm taking the medication, I notice it has no refills, and I begin to worry. What if I take all the pills and I'm still nauseous?

I decide to call the pharmacy at Zangmeister. I learn that if I need additional nausea medication that all I need to do is call for a refill. The pharmacist does let me know that they close at noon on Friday, but if I need anything that day they can always call it in to my local pharmacy.

However, when I ask him about whether or not I should expect an energy drop when I stop taking Prednisone, and whether there is anything I can do to prepare for that, he tells me that he's never heard anyone complain of that before and doesn't think I should expect a problem. I hope he's right, but I'm concerned about what I might encounter when I stop taking it.

By the second day after getting chemo my taste is off and nothing tastes right. Even my favorite raspberry lemonade tastes too strong and seems to irritate the inside of my mouth. Later my mouth starts getting really sore inside. I have excellent dental hygiene with very strong gums, so I'm surprised when flossing hurts my gums, my electric toothbrushes hurt my gums and my mouthwash actually feels like it's burning the inside of my mouth. My first step is to stop flossing, stop using my electric toothbrushes and stop using the regular mouthwash. I switch to just using soft bristle toothbrushes instead. That helps, but I worry about what is happening to me.

It gets worse. Now I have a sore on my lip, inside and out and sore spots on the right side on my tongue. I don't want to drink anything, the opposite of what I'm supposed to be doing. I have Carmex, something I've used in the past that worked when I had a fever blister, but since I haven't had one for a very long time, it takes me a while to find an unopened container.

With the soreness in my mouth I try other drinks ... fresh lemonade ... but the citrus stings my mouth. The same thing happens with just hot lemon water. I'm atypical and don't care very much for tea. My daughter recommends diluting my raspberry lemonade to see if that helps make it easier to drink. And it does. It takes about a 50% reduction in strength to make it drinkable without hurting me. I also load up on no sugar added fruit popsicles. This is another way to get fluid inside my body when I'm having trouble drinking as much as I need.

The Carmex for my lip sores isn't working, in fact it seems to make my lips drier, even splitting, and more painful. I don't even feel well enough to get dressed, let alone go to the store, so my daughter Suzanne offers to get a different product for my dry lips and something for the sores on my lip. The Chapstick she selects to soothe my lips is very firm, almost too firm to use on my tender lips.

My mouth is deteriorating I can tell. My gums are swollen and hurt so much they are causing my teeth to hurt. I'm really scared at this point and don't know what to do for myself. I decide it's time to call the doctor.

The call is answered in the nurse's station right away, and I begin, "Hi, this is Carol Rosebrough, and I had my first chemo treatment on Monday. I'm having a lot of trouble with side effects and I need help."

"Oh, hi Carol, this is Kenya; I remember you ... I was the one who gave you your Neulasta shot on Tuesday. How can I help you?"

I'm so relieved to hear Kenya's cheerful and welcoming voice, I'm nearly moved to tears. And I feel special that she remembers me. She's made me feel safe enough to begin explaining all my symptoms to her. She hears me and understands. She thinks a magic mouthwash will help me. She says she'll check with the doctor and call me back. When she calls me back within the hour, I learn she has already called in the prescription to my local pharmacy. She asks that I give them a little time to make up the mouthwash since they have to mix several different ingredients together. She tells me to call back if I need anything else. It's a wonderful exchange and I'm grateful she's working in that area today. My fears subside.

The "Magic Mouthwash" is exactly what she said. Magic. It's a pink kind of thick liquid that has four different ingredients. It's odd to use and I don't really like it, but I use it. I'm only to use one or two teaspoons at a time, and I wonder how such a small amount can be effective. But it is. It doesn't take very long for my mouth to heal. Within days my mouth and gums have healed enough that I'm able to floss and use my electric toothbrushes again.

The Abreva Suzanne selected for the sores on my lip works great, but then I begin to get some pimple like sores on my face. I just use the Abreva on those as well, and all of them heal pretty quickly. Unfortunately my lips remain tender and the firm Chapstick is difficult to apply without hurting me. Again, my daughter searches for an alternative and she chooses Aquaphor, a lip repair, and it works beautifully. It's very soft and easy to apply on my tender lips. It keeps my lips moist and they begin to heal as well.

For several days I haven't had very much to drink. Between the treatment, medications and sore mouth, I'm bloated, my stomach hurts and I'm constipated. I know that a lot of the constipation and bloating is my own fault for not being able to drink enough and food losing its taste.

And then, one more side effect hits me a week after treatment. At about midnight I start having pain, actually a throbbing, pulsating pain. It seems to be concentrated in my upper arms and my lower back. And I have a tightness in my chest.

I'm scared. *What is happening? Is this a stroke? Am I having a heart attack?* I've already had one warning stroke, and if this is another one, it could be much more serious. I try several positions to see if it will alleviate the pain, but nothing works. It's like something inside me is pounding, pulsating and it's so painful. What should I do? Should I try to call Zangmeister? Should I call 911? Again, I keep moving, trying to get comfortable or to lessen the pain, but nothing is working. However, since the pain is in my upper arms and lower back it doesn't make sense I could be having a stroke or heart attack.

I decide to get up and take two Tylenol first to see what happens. If the pain continues, then I'll call someone. Fortunately the Tylenol does help and it calms my body. Of course my mind can't stop thinking about what is happening, so I don't sleep, but at least my body has a chance to rest. I'm still confused though about what caused this pain and know I need to report this reaction tomorrow to Dr. Patel.

When I talk to my daughter Suzanne the next morning, she thinks it's a reaction to the Neulasta shot. She reminds me I was told the Neulasta works in my bone marrow making and pumping out new white blood cells and I could have a side effect of muscle and bone pain from it. Since the pain finally stopped after I took the Tylenol, I think that must be the cause after all.

That morning I call Zangmeister to report this side effect that I had during the night and again, Kenya is working the desk. I'm grateful to have her cheerful and calm assistance. I tell her the symptoms and what I think it is. She tends to think it's not a reaction to the Neulasta since it's been days since I had the shot, and she's never heard of such a reaction before. But she agrees to check with Dr. Patel and call me back. When she calls me back, I learn that Dr. Patel agrees with me. He, too, thinks it's a side effect to the Neulasta shot. Now I know for sure I wasn't having a stroke or a heart attack and for that I'm much relieved and grateful. Fortunately I have no recurrence of this symptom.

I have one other side effect following this first chemo treatment, but it isn't due to the chemo. It's from the excessive washing of my hands. I didn't realize how many times I should wash my hands, but now I do, and my hands are raw, dry and cracking. Regular hand lotion doesn't even phase it.

My younger daughter Rebecca, who lives in the MD/DC area suggests using coconut oil to heal my hands. My daughter Suzanne gives me a small container to try, to make sure it works for me before buying some. She also suggests using a plastic spoon to take a portion of the solid coconut oil from the container to use. That way I'll not leave any skin cells behind in the container to possibly yield any bacteria later.

The coconut oil is a fabulous solution, and the healing of my hands begins almost immediately. I keep a container of the coconut oil and plastic spoons in the kitchen and in my master bathroom. My hands heal rather quickly, and I'm thrilled with the solution.

I also change my body lotion to a fragrance free one with a little more density than the one I previously used. I completely coat my body with this Curel lotion immediately after every shower, every day. It helps to keep my skin moist. I continue to use my facial moisturizer on my face every day as well.

I also replace the liquid antibiotic hand soap in the bathrooms and kitchen soap dispensers with a liquid Ivory soap. The regular antibiotic soap seemed to be too harsh for my tender skin. The softer Ivory soap definitely helps lessen the negative impact of the excessive washing.

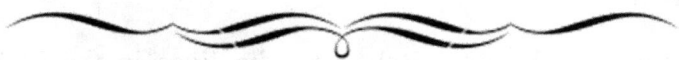

I believe at the darkest hour,

the greatest light emerges

and a new path is revealed.

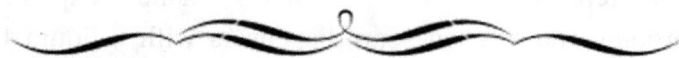

Chapter 7

My Second Treatment

By the time I reach the third week after my first treatment, I start feeling normal for the first time since starting chemo, and I love it. I begin to think that chemotherapy may not be so bad after all. I'm well enough to do the sanitizing around the house and to change my bed linens the night before my second treatment.

I prepare three containers of my Crystal Light raspberry lemonade to take with me for this second treatment, and I have plenty of nutritious finger food to last the day. I have my low sodium peanut butter and blackberry jelly sandwich on wheat bread, cut into quarters, a boiled egg with pepper, grapes, an apple cored, skin on and cut into quarters, saltine crackers with unsalted tops, ginger snap cookies, chocolate pudding and a granola bar. If I get nauseous during treatment, the crackers will be a big help. I know I have more food than I can possibly eat during the day, but since I'm literally trapped during treatment, and will be there all day, I want to have everything I might possibly want to eat and drink while there.

I feel ready. I can't find my sleep mask anywhere, so I pack a dry wash cloth to cover my eyes during treatment. I also pack a light pair of gloves to keep my hands warm during treatment. Even with the three warm blankets given to me during the first treatment, I still couldn't seem to get my hands warm.

I've done everything I can think of to take care of myself and to prevent infection. Knowing that I may not feel well for a few days after treatment, I have food ready for easy preparation and the house will not need anything done right away. I can stay in bed for days if I need to do so. Hopefully my side effects from this second treatment will not be as severe as the ones from the first treatment.

My meeting with Dr. Patel begins with him asking me to tell him about my side effects from the first treatment and I begin the litany, step by step, of everything that occurred.

When I've finished, he somberly says he plans to reduce the chemo drug by 20% or I'll end up in the hospital. I am pretty shocked by this thought. He then adds that the chemo has a cumulative effect on the body and the initial dose is based on height and weight, but it can be adjusted.

He also is thinking of eliminating the Neulasta shot because of the side effects I had. But now I worry I've complained too much about the side effects. The Neulasta shot builds white blood cells and that is a great help for me to fight infections.

"Dr. Patel, I only had that pounding pain one night, I'm not sure you need to discontinue this booster shot just because of that. If that's the only side effect I have, I don't mind it now that I know what's happening."

"Okay, Carol. The Neulasta shot isn't like the chemo, it isn't cumulative in the body, in fact the effects get less with each treatment. We'll continue it."

He has one other suggestion for me. When I tell him about the problem with my hands due to excessive washing, he recommends cocoa butter instead of the coconut oil I've been using. I agree to try it.

When I arrive on the second floor for the chemo infusion, I'm approached by the nurse saying that I'll be in her pod today. When I realize this is a station in the back of the room, I hesitate a second and then tell her I want to be seated by the window wall. She says I have been assigned to her pod for the day, and can't change it.

I don't like this arrangement. The seat assigned to me has two seats facing me on the other side of this section, one positioned slightly to my left and one to my right. I'll no longer have the privacy and the tree line view that I had for my first treatment. And two patients will be in my view the entire day. Now I'm really glad I brought the wash cloth with me to cover my eyes. Unfortunately I didn't bring any music to listen to during the day. I won't make that mistake next time.

The wash cloth gives me the privacy I crave and blocks the overhead florescent lights, but I can't seem to block out the chatting that goes on during the day. I was scared before coming for this treatment, and my blood pressure was higher than normal when they checked my vitals beforehand. I feel added stress by not being able to relax while the chemo drugs are entering my body.

I know it's important for me to relax and bless the drugs as they do their job to heal me, but I seem agitated and unable to calm myself. I meditate and that helps short term, but I never achieve the calmness that would benefit me the most. I decide right then and there I will bring music to listen to the next time and buy a real sleep mask. The wash cloth works, but it continually slips down my face, again causing agitation with the necessity to move it back in place over and over again.

I get through the day and the nurse hugs me at the end telling me what a great job I've done during the day. I think I must have just grunted at her knowing that it wasn't an easy day for me. I leave deciding I'll specifically request a seat by the window wall for my next treatment.

The infusion took about an hour less time this visit. I was able to tolerate a faster speed of the drugs entering my body. My daughter Suzanne brought me to this visit as well, and again she stayed for the entire day. Getting on the highway just that hour earlier means less traffic getting home. I'm grateful to be home and am prepared to stay in bed watching movies. Suzanne has loaned me six seasons of Doc Martin to watch.

Chapter 8

Grieving Cancer Diagnosis

I think it's impossible to receive a cancer diagnosis without having some sort of emotional reaction. It's one of those life changing moments. I went through a sped up version of the grieving process before being able to settle down into a level of acceptance of what I'm going through.

My first reaction was shock. I was so unprepared for such a diagnosis. After the warning stroke last year, I have eaten nutritionally, exercised and taken really great care of myself. And in the process I slowly and naturally lost more than 50 pounds. With my health and energy improving, I just didn't believe I could possibly have cancer ... now.

Unfortunately my denial didn't last very long. I couldn't maintain my denial when I received confirmation that I did indeed have cancer and chemotherapy was the recommended treatment.

But then I became angry. I've been living a spiritual life for decades, hurting no one, healing the wounds of my past and forgiving my abusers. And for the past year turning my life around to take care of myself and love my body. Why do I need cancer? I've already given up fast food, soda, caffeine, salt, potato chips, ice cream, my favorite foods. What on earth is my lesson in having cancer? It didn't seem fair.

But grief will have its way whether it's dealt with in the moment or postponed until some future date. If it was possible, I knew it would be best to honor my grief about having cancer and work through all the feelings that came up. The more processing I could do now, the faster I would move through the grief and get on to living my life ... even during the time I'm having chemotherapy.

The answer to my question about what is my lesson, is really twofold. First, I've been in denial of my body my entire life, at least until a year ago when I had the warning stroke. When I lost the right side of my body, only for moments, it got my attention like nothing ever could. I saw so clearly that I needed my body and my body needed me to take care of it.

It's not as though I hated my body all my life, it was as though it didn't exist. I understand how ridiculous that might sound, but it's true. I was sexually molested the first time by a neighbor when I was five years old and then later by another neighbor. My father raged at and verbally and sexually abused my mother. Even though my father never turned his rage on me, I never felt loved or safe in my own home. I learned early in life how to live in denial of my surroundings and my body.

And then when I was 14 years old, my mother died of leukemia and I moved in with my older sister and her family. I was very happy with this decision because I thought my sister cared about me. My sister worked in her own family's business plus she kept the books for my father's coal mine. My sister was very nice, and my brother-in-law talked to me, which no one else ever did. I thought for sure my life would be improved living with them.

What I didn't know is that my sister pressured my dad to let me live with her and for her to become my legal guardian. She knew I had a steady boyfriend and she convinced my dad I was headed for trouble because he couldn't possibly watch out for me like she could. My dad trusted my sister and he always listened to her.

But I don't think it really was her idea for me to move in with them. I think it was my brother-in-law's idea, and he convinced my sister it was what would be best for me. It was when he offered me a ride in his car, asking me if anything sexual was happening with my boyfriend, Jack, that I believe his plan was conceived. In my naiveté, I didn't even realize it was inappropriate for him to be asking me these questions. I wish I had had the presence of mind to lie to him, but I didn't. I told him we were petting, but that was all.

He looked upset with me and I knew that I was in trouble. I just could not possibly know how it would play out. After I moved in with my sister, my brother-in-law told me I was no longer allowed to date Jack. I was filled with despair at the thought of not being able to see him again. How could this be? The only person I had ever known who seemed to really like me and now I couldn't even see him?

I was desperate. Sobbing, I begged my brother-in-law to change his mind. I said I would do anything if he would allow me to continue to see Jack. *Gotcha!* My brother-in-law agreed ... with conditions. I had to be home by 11 PM, and I would be docked from my allowance for every five minutes I was late. I also had to double date, to ensure that Jack and I would not be alone, and have an inspection after every date to prove I was still a virgin. Wait ... What? An inspection?? What did that even mean???

I didn't know what to do. All I knew was I couldn't stand the thought of not seeing Jack. I agreed to the terms of the deal with no way of knowing the lifelong impact this decision would have on my body.

The inspections were quite like a gynecological vaginal exam. I became even more disassociated from my body than ever during these inspections and I learned to escape my body when they took place. I didn't acknowledge my body at all, it was as though it just disappeared. Because these inspections were based on the fact I couldn't be trusted, (according to my brother-in-law) and that sex outside marriage was bad, all sorts of other psychological problems were implanted within me that took years to unravel.

After a lifetime of not acknowledging my body, the stroke a year ago jolted me awake to my body, and how desperately it needed me to take care of it. Most of my life I was thin and food was not an issue for me. However, when I was 49, I quit smoking and unconsciously started using food instead. Food tasted so much better to me after I quit smoking, but since I had never had a weight problem, I didn't realize I needed to limit myself. I gained a lot of weight quickly.

Because I was still in such denial of my body at that time, I never acknowledged the weight gain, and I carried it up until the time I had the stroke. When I was heavy, doctors told me I had high cholesterol and high blood pressure and needed medications for both these conditions, but it didn't make any difference in my behavior. I changed nothing at the time, except to start taking the medications they prescribed.

But I did change when I had the stroke. What happened to me I am not certain. I just know the denial about my body evaporated and I became obsessed with figuring out what my body needed and how I could help my body become healthy.

I wrote an affirmation just a few weeks after the stroke and typed it in extremely large bold and italic letters, printed it, signed it, dated it, put it on cardboard and placed it standing up on my desk so that I could see it from any direction. Following is the affirmation:

I am in excellent health

with a

very fit, strong and

flexible body !!

In addition to this affirmation posted visibly on my desk, I began to write it every day in my journal. I wrote it over and over again, like a mantra, declaring it as a current fact so that

I could believe it in every fiber of my being and do everything possible to make it so.

And it happened. During this past year I lost over 50 pounds. Not with any gimmicks or eliminating any food groups, but with going to a very nutritious, mostly plant based diet with portion control, counting caloric intake and giving up fast food, soda, salt, high fat, caffeine, potato chips and ice cream.

I have always had excellent personal hygiene for the exterior of my body, but prior to this time I never took notice of what I put into my body, or even what was happening inside there. I was literally numb to the effect of how what I put into my body could hurt it. Now I wanted to educate myself. With a lifetime of junk food, fast food, convenience packaged foods and eating on the go between meetings for work, it was probably an insurmountable task to make a complete life change at my age, but I did.

I've tried changing my eating habits in the past, but after the stroke it was different. I wasn't making this change for anyone else, or because anyone else was putting pressure on me to do it. I was making this change to take care of my body and to help it get healthy, and I knew whatever changes I made needed to be permanent. I researched food and nutrition and calories on the Internet. The U.S. Department of Agriculture actually has wonderful information on the Internet about healthy eating, and I decided this was how I wanted to eat. I wanted to give my body what it needed to work well, and I wanted to put less into my body so it didn't have to work so hard.

In meditation I visualized the fatty deposits in my body melting and leaving my body effortlessly daily through my waste. Nothing happened overnight, but the .2 to .4 pound loss per day added up. And losing it very slowly meant no trauma for my body to overcome. Just a gradual, slow process with good food coming in to help my body do its job. I was in no hurry. This was a permanent life style change.

I decided to make short term weight loss goals for myself. Again, something I could sign and post on my desk. I settled on a two week time period with a two pound loss goal for the two weeks. I used 3 x 5 index cards, dated, putting my current weight, the new goal weight and target date. The few other times when I made attempts at weight loss, just for the sake of weight loss, I would get to the 200 pound level and then boomerang back to where I was or higher. I knew there must be some sense of protection with this weight level that I had to process, or I would never be successful at helping my body become healthy. I decided to ask my body for permission to pass through to my next weight loss goal. I continued asking permission with every weight loss goal, even long after I passed through the 200 pound mark on my way down. I signed each card and taped it to my printer. I weighed myself every morning and logged my weight on the computer to make sure I stayed on target to meet or exceed my goal. At the end of the two week period, I wrote my current weight, noting if I had met or exceeded my goal and again signed my name. I started my next two week goal with this ending weight. I kept all the cards.

Because I was unfamiliar with food quantity and calories, I also needed an education in how to monitor what I was eating. I found a great website for calories and full ingredient content of every kind of food. Again, using 3 x 5 cards, I started collecting not only calorie counts of specific foods, but also the full caloric ingredient content of everything I put into my body. Until I had the catalog of cards, I needed to take the individual foods into my office and log their caloric ingredients directly from the food, or check the fresh food content on the website. Next I developed an Excel spread sheet and tracked all the caloric ingredients of everything I ate and the total for each day.

When I started this new eating plan, I read that I should never fall below 1200 calories per day or I would risk going into starvation mode and have a backlash craving food, and possibly a binge. My daughter Suzanne also cautioned me to make sure I maintained at least 1200 calories per day. I found this very tricky to do, but I worked at it. It seemed that my most consistent weight loss happened if I stayed between 1200 and 1300 calories. Much over that I either stayed flat or I gained. I had never done anything like this in my life, but I accepted it and approached it as though taking on a new job. And this new job was taking care of my body to the best of my ability.

I came to the conclusion that the warning stroke I had was just that. It was a warning that if I did not change how I was treating and feeding my body, that the next warning would be much stronger and cause actual damage to my body. I spent three days in the hospital after I had this warning stroke, and felt very weak at first, but I had no lasting damage. I knew I would not be so lucky if I had another one. Of course, a major stroke could also take my life away from me completely.

For an entire year I stayed on this eating plan and I also added exercising. I walked my dog, Buddy, once or twice a day and I used free weights every other day. It truly felt like I was in training and it was working. Slowly but surely, my energy increased and the weight kept coming off. Eating well was becoming easier as I learned new ways to cook for myself and I started to enjoy eating fresh fruits and vegetables every day. I had worked for over 34 years straight building a career and never felt very domestic, so I found myself pleasantly surprised not only that I could do this, but that I was actually enjoying doing it.

And just weeks before I received my cancer diagnosis the first real evidence of my healing presented itself. I no longer needed medication to control blood pressure! Eliminating salt from my diet and reducing my food intake to only what my body needed was producing concrete healthy results for my body.

So, why cancer now? It didn't seem fair since I had already gotten the message to love my body and take care of it with the warning stroke. But then I learned that the cancer was there first, long before the stroke. And having the stroke first basically got me stronger and ready to do all the things I needed to do to take care of myself while healing from cancer.

I began to think my affirmation of having excellent health brought the cancer to my attention. It was there growing for years before it was discovered, and it was only discovered after I started using the affirmation that I'm in excellent health. One can't have excellent health while having incurable slow growing cancer somewhere in the body. And it was while I was getting to know my body I discovered the lump under my left eyelid.

During this same time, I was experiencing intermittent double vision. I had been attributing it to the stroke since Dr. Barfield, my neurologist, had told me it was the vision part of my brain that was affected by the stroke. Oddly enough it was this double vision that prompted Dr. Sparling to refer me to Dr. Calloway. And it was when he referred me to Dr. Gallo that I actually learned the lump under my left eyelid was cancer.

So why couldn't I just have a few treatments of radiation and be done with it? To save my eyesight of course. It has all worked out to be just as it should be. I have no doubt I will have my excellent health and very fit, strong and flexible body when I am finished healing and am cancer free.

I accept that I have cancer now. I'm not angry or blaming my body or the cancer. It is what it is. Now it's up to me to do everything I can to manage my life and help my body get through this with the best chance of a positive outcome. I'm talking to my body. I'm apologizing to my body. I know it's not my body's fault this has happened. I'm apologizing to my body for not listening all these years and overeating and eating wrong things and eating too late so that it has to work hard all night digesting food. I started a year ago to take care of the inside of my body for the first time in my life, and now I promise to take care of my body and treasure it the rest of my days. We are partners now. We need each other. And it's truly a matter of our partnership being until death do us part.

I no longer count every calorie and log it every day. After a year of this intense concentration I've learned what portions are and what I need to eat to keep my body operating at optimal health. I'll continue for the rest of my life eating a low sodium, low fat diet with foods as close to their natural state as possible. Portion control can help me maintain the weight loss that has already occurred so that I can end my cancer treatment at the same weight as I started. My concern during this chemotherapy treatment is to eat nutritiously and stay as healthy as possible. Weight maintenance is my goal during treatment, rather than weight loss.

This is not as simple as it sounds. With every chemotherapy treatment, I gain about five pounds just from all the liquid infusions into my body. Although I'm not on a weight loss plan during therapy, I have to be cognizant of this weight gain and make sure I lose it before the next treatment cycle. If I don't monitor my food intake, especially right after treatment, that weight doesn't come off. And that is what happened after my second chemo treatment. I consider using my 3 x 5 cards again just for this purpose.

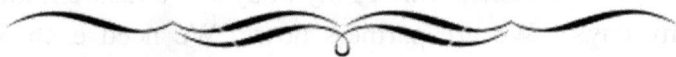

I believe every day is a gift and

an opportunity

to forgive, heal and grow

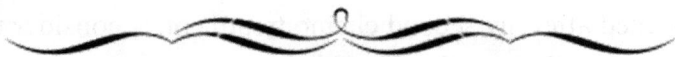

Chapter 9

My Third Chemo Treatment

Knowing that the first day or so following chemotherapy I'm most at risk for an infection, I'm diligent in sanitizing the house again prior to this treatment. My bed is changed, I've sanitized my CPAP equipment and bathrooms, plus all the light switches, door knobs, cabinet handles, computer keys, remotes, DVD player, toothbrush handles, soap dispenser handles, hair brush ... anything my hands touch, I want to sanitize.

I prepare most of my food and drinks to take with me on treatment day the evening before, except for the peanut butter and jelly sandwich, which I save to make in the morning. I'm taking a big salad to eat during this treatment and hope that it will be easy enough for me to eat in the chemo infusion chair. This time I have a real sleep mask, with an adjustable strap, to wear during the day, I've packed my gloves, CD player and Walkman plus CDs and cassettes to listen to during the day. I'm ready.

When I meet with Dr. Patel, the first thing he asks me about are my side effects. I tell him about the flushing and chest pain I experienced and he reduces my Prednisone medication from four pills a day to three, but I'm still to take them for the five days after treatment, the same as before. I'm grateful for the reduced dosage and hope it also reduces my level of hyper activity.

He notices my weight gain on the chart and comments that I must be eating very well. I explain to him that the weight gain is from the last chemo treatment and that I've been eating very nutritious food. He tells me that the weight gain from a chemo treatment is just from the fluid intake and that it should come off. I do acknowledge that I've been overeating, although with all good food, and that is why the chemo added weight never came off.

The most important news of the day is learning that my fourth chemo treatment will be delayed one week. Instead, I'll have another PET body scan to check the extent of my cancer remaining. That scan will determine if the chemo treatment is working to heal the cancer, or if treatment needs to be changed in some way.

On the one hand I'll find out how much cancer the chemotherapy drugs have removed from my body. However, my mind quickly leaps to the "what if" scenario. *What if it isn't working as they intended or expected? If treatment needs to change, will I have to go through new side effects as though I'm just beginning chemotherapy?*

Next stop, the chemo infusion room. When I arrive I'm told that I'll be seated in the same section where I was for the second treatment. I'm not happy. I tell the nurse I've requested a seat by the window wall. She acknowledges that my request is on my chart, but that she has been assigned to care for me and she can't possibly see me or take care of me well if I'm that far away. I start to object, but realize I'm prepared for this. I'm seated on the other side of the area where I was last time, which somehow seems much better for me. Plus I have my sleep mask and my music if I do indeed need a distraction to stay relaxed.

The chatter is less on this visit, and my preparation is paying off. My blood pressure was normal for this visit for the first time since I started chemo. With the sleep mask and the music I'm able to fully relax, meditate and I actually fall asleep during a good part of the day.

Later in the day, the nurse tells me others saw my mask and said they were going to get one, too. And while I was eating my lovely salad of spinach, romaine and green leaf lettuce with grape tomatoes and cauliflower, a couple of people passing by commented on how good it looked. It was delicious and easy to eat while I was getting my chemo treatment, so I decide to take a salad for all my other visits.

The day passes quickly and I learn that the time needed was less again, nearly an hour less. I think I'm at the maximum speed for the infusion now. The ride home seems effortless and we encounter no rush hour traffic on the highway.

I have more side effects after this treatment. The flushing (a redness and very hot feeling in my face) that I had after the second treatment starts this time on the day after treatment. I take the Benedryl that was successful to stop the flushing before, but this time it doesn't seem to make any difference. By the next morning the flushing seems to be worse and I'm afraid to take any more Prednisone. I decide to call

Zangmeister to ask what I should do. I'm told to stop taking the Prednisone. It works. The flushing fades and doesn't return.

The next side effect is my scalp. It's itching and I find myself scratching my head during the night. Little bumps, sore to the touch, are also appearing. However, I'm not experiencing as much overall soreness and tenderness as I had after the second treatment. I call Zangmeister to ask what I should do and if I should change to a medicated shampoo. When I don't get my normal call back right away, I decide to call Dr. Nixon, my dermatologist. Fortunately she has a cancellation and I can see her right away. She checks my scalp and tells me that my reaction is minimal and could be coming from the cancer or the treatment. She prescribes two liquid medications to apply to my scalp daily and thinks I don't need to change shampoos.

However, my dandruff shampoo is stinging my scalp now, so I search for an alternative to use for the short term. I find a product I have never heard of or noticed before. It is Clear ... Scalp and Hair. The description on the product says it is nourishing to the scalp ... just what I need. I bought the shampoo and conditioner and miracle of all miracles, they work. My scalp doesn't sting when I use either one. Between my change in shampoo and conditioner and the medication from Dr. Nixon, my scalp heals and the scalp problems do not return.

It's definitely not surprising to have scalp issues during chemotherapy treatment. Chemo drugs attack cancer cells which are fast growing cells. Unfortunately hair follicle cells are also fast growing and the drugs attack those as well. No wonder people lose hair and the scalp can become quite sore, tender and even get sores on it!

I decide it's time to write, print, sign, date and post an affirmation that my cancer is totally and completely healed. The following one is posted in my office, right above my computer.

My cancer is

totally and completely

healed

now and

forevermore !!

I believe when I don't get

the lesson at a subtle level,

the lesson will keep appearing in some form

with stronger and stronger levels

until I do.

Chapter 10

Mid-Way PET Scan Testing

Today is my scheduled PET body scan, which will reveal how successful the treatment has been in reducing my cancer so far. I'm a bit nervous actually. I thought this testing would be done when I was finished with chemotherapy, not in the middle of treatment.

Of course it's a great idea not to wait until the end. It will give the opportunity to adjust the chemo drugs if the tumor is not responding as expected. On the one hand I am grateful that the testing is being done now, and yet on the other hand I wonder what will happen if it isn't responding as well as expected. Plus, I have been affirming that the cancer is being cleared away. The extra test somehow puts doubt in my mind. And that I need to clear away.

What I noticed, when I started chemotherapy, was that my eyes weren't level. The tumor, which was under my left eye, had grown so large that it tilted my eye upward. When looking straight at my eyes in the mirror, it was possible to visibly see they were not on the same level!

After I had the warning stroke, Dr. Barfield showed me the MRI (Magnetic Resonance Imaging) from the hospital and pointed out the little white spots of damage in the vision part of my brain. At that time, it seemed logical to me that this damage was the root cause of my double vision.

I was terrified the first time I had vision problems while I was driving. I was on a two lane road, only a mile and a half from my home. All of a sudden I saw multiple lanes and cars and couldn't tell what was real. I pulled off the road immediately and parked on the shoulder with my emergency lights flashing. I had no idea how in the world I could possibly drive the rest of the way home safely.

It took a while to calm down, but then I discovered if I adjusted my glasses, tilting one side up higher than the other, then I could see clearly again. Not knowing why this helped at the time, I thought I might be able to drive the short distance home. Unfortunately I had to keep holding my glasses in a tilt with my right hand and steer with my left. If I let go of the glasses, or even let them shift from that one position then the multiple images returned.

Now it all makes sense. My vision problems were a result of the lump under my left eye tilting my left eye upward. When I tilted my glasses, it literally put my eyes at the same level and restored my normal vision! Even though I knew I could correct my vision when problems occurred, I remained very cautious and only drove short distances. Once the lump under my eye was gone, I had no recurrence of any vision problems.

Since I can't feel the tumor any longer when I touch my eye lid, and my vision is restored with no setbacks of multiple images, there has to be quite an improvement in the extent of the tumor under my eye. I wonder ... could the cancer be completely gone already? Wouldn't that be wonderful? But now I have the waiting game. First the tests, and the waiting to hear the results and what happens next.

My appointment for the scan is not until 9:15 AM today, and it requires fasting beforehand. It takes nearly an hour to drive to Zangmeister and the testing will last two hours. I know I need to pack drinks and food to have as soon as the test is over. Now that I have a commitment not to eat fast food or drink soda, I don't want to leave home without being prepared. Being away from home for such a long time, and hungry, or thirsty, is way too much temptation for me to stay away from fast food, and I am determined to honor my commitment. I pack my standard peanut butter and jelly sandwich, a fruit salad with fresh strawberries, blueberries, grapes and bananas, wheat crackers and red pepper hummus and two containers of my raspberry lemonade. I am ready. I will not be tempted.

I had this same scan prior to beginning chemotherapy, but I totally forgot everything except being in the tube. Now I remember the first hour is all preparation for the PET scan. The first step is to insert an IV in my arm, and the nurse is great. She gets it into my vein on the first try! To most people that may not seem like such an accomplishment, but to me it is fantastic. My veins are very small and deep. In the past, there have been times that a nurse needed up to three attempts before getting a needle inserted into my vein correctly to draw blood or to insert an IV, and on some occasions even needing to call in a different nurse to get it right!

I am in a small room with a large leather lounge chair. There is a small tray extension on each side. The IV is in my right arm, the nurse excuses herself and comes back carrying a metal container that has a handle in the middle. She puts it down on the cabinet that is close to the door. The container has the radiation that will be inserted into the IV.

The middle of the container is all that is removed. My nurse gently carries this portion of the container with an extension arm to the table by my right arm. She explains it is a small amount of radiation and will not harm me. Of course she has gloves on, but she has to remove one piece from the container which exposes the needle. That needle is what she inserts into the IV. Once the radiation is in my body, she closes that part of the container back onto the needle, and puts the container back together. It looks something like a miniature metal rocket. Then she inserts a syringe of saline solution into the IV to make sure it is cleaned out. Then this part is over.

A cotton ball is placed on the part of my arm where the needle was inserted and then it is wrapped with some kind of stretchy material to put pressure on the area.

The next stage is to drink a liquid. I'm not sure of the function, but I think it is to help things show up on the scan. I have chosen the flavor of raspberry to make the drink a little more palatable. After I drink this liquid, I need to wait for 45 minutes, then I will drink the same amount again and wait 15 minutes. Then I will have the scan.

Since I have total privacy in this room, I ask that all the lights be turned off. And I am cold. I tend to get cold when I'm nervous, plus the room seems quite cold. The nurse gets me a warm blanket, turns on a room heater and I put on my jacket and gloves. I'm toasty warm, the room is dark, it is quiet, and I fully relax while these drugs go through my body. I breathe deeply, I relax even further. I say my mantra, *The Lord's Prayer* over and over. And then the strangest thing happens. The tune from *South Pacific* "I'm Gonna Wash That Man Right Outa My Hair" comes into my mind, but with slightly different words.

This is the song I heard:

"I'm gonna wash that cancer right out of me, I'm gonna wash that cancer right out of me, I'm gonna wash that cancer right out of me and send it on its way!"

The song's tune is cheerful, it is positive and actually empowering. It gives me a sense of taking charge, and being in charge of the cancer.

With this tune in my head, I cheerfully leave the privacy of my quiet room and head toward the room with the tube machine. It will provide the status of how much cancer is in my body and where. This room seems really cold to me, and because I can't wear anything metal in this machine, I can't wear my jacket. It has a metal zipper. Again, the nurse provides me with a warm blanket and I ask for my gloves to keep my hands warm. I have to have my arms above my head so I am grateful I'm wearing a long-sleeved shirt and that I have my gloves to wear. With the blanket, I will be warm enough.

I am inside this tube machine for a half hour or so, and surprisingly the time passes pretty quickly. I close my eyes and breathe to help myself relax. It's not easy for me to be still and not move a muscle for such a long time, but today it doesn't seem difficult. I keep thinking about the tune in my head, washing the cancer out of me and sending it on its way and visioning that it is completely gone from my body.

It seems no time at all when I am told I'm all done. The table moves to take me out of the machine and I try to lift my arms. I've been still so long in an unfamiliar position, my arms seem frozen in position! I ask the nurse to help me. We both laugh a bit and once she begins to lift my arms, I am okay. I do have to sit on the side of the table a couple of minutes, just to get my bearings. Before I leave this area, I receive a card stating I am radioactive! I will need it if I am passing through any security as I will set off the alarms for the next two to three days!

My daughter Suzanne is waiting for me. While she has a conversation with my grandson on her cell phone before we start the drive home, I begin to eat my food in the car. Everything I have lovingly prepared for myself to have today is quite delicious, especially the fresh fruit and hummus. Other than the "special" drink I had for the test, I've had nothing to drink or eat since about 6 PM yesterday. I'm so thirsty I literally guzzle the raspberry lemonade.

With our trip home being mid-day, traffic is very light and I am feeling very light myself. It is a good day, and I am grateful.

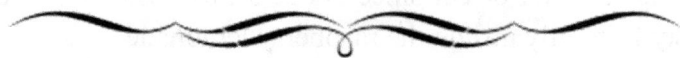

I believe a shift in inner perception

changes everything else even when no

outward change happens.

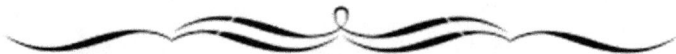

Chapter 11

Loving My Body

Prior to August of last year, my body was a literal non-entity to me. I gave it no thought or care, other than to keep the exterior of me clean and to wear clean clothes every day. Not once, in my entire life, did I really give a thought about what I was putting into my body. A couple of times, when I was early in my spiritual seeking, I did try to eat a healthier diet. But that was always someone else's idea, and with the lack of connection to my body, the change never lasted and I went back to my life-long habit of fast food, junk food and soda.

However, on that fateful day last August, I had a stroke. I was lucky. It was called a warning stroke, a TIA (Transient Ischemic Attack). I had no lasting damage. But, for a few moments, I lost the feeling and use of my entire right side.

Moments before the stroke happened, I had just left my office to walk into the kitchen and I was near the counter closest to my office. Without any warning, the room started spinning and I felt extremely dizzy. I thought for sure I was going to pass out and collapse on the floor. Everything happened instantaneously. All I knew was I had to keep myself from falling on the floor. Not knowing the feeling was already gone from the right side of my body, I thought I could grab onto or lean on the countertop with my right arm, but I had already started to fall. Instead of being able to grab onto the countertop, my upper right arm and shoulder slammed into the edge of the granite countertop full force. I heard the thud of the impact, but I felt no pain. As that happened, I had the presence of mind to use my left arm to hang onto an open lower cabinet door to keep from falling completely onto the floor. I knew something was terribly wrong with my body, but I wasn't sure what was happening.

As I was slumped over the door, clinging to it for dear life, I looked at my right side. My arm hung limply at my side. When I poked it with my left hand, it just moved back and forth slowly on its own and I couldn't feel anything when I touched it ... it was completely numb. In absolute panic it occurred to me ... *I'm having a stroke!*

It was the most frightening experience of my life. Immediately I went into shock. How badly I had neglected and unconsciously abused my body my entire life flashed before my eyes in those first few seconds. It became crystal clear that I was nothing without my body, and that my body needed me to take care of it. I was filled with remorse and regret that it had taken a stroke and 73 years, two months and five days of living for me to "get it".

Fortunately I never lost consciousness. I started screaming at the top of my lungs for my son, John, who was asleep upstairs, and I kept screaming until I could hear him running down the stairs. As soon as he saw me, he called 911 and then helped me back into my office onto my desk chair. I sat there until the emergency crew arrived just minutes later.

Shortly after they arrived, they asked me what happened, took my vitals, then helped me onto a stretcher. All the way to the hospital emergency room, the EMTs talked to me, and asked me to focus my eyes on them. They kept asking me questions doing their best to keep me conscious, and it worked. I never lost consciousness during any part of the stroke.

The hospital performed tests, including an MRI. The doctor on call confirmed I had a stroke and I was admitted. While there, I had such a splitting headache in the back of my head I thought it would explode. The feeling that I lost on my right side during the stroke came back entirely, but I still felt very weak. Later, when I moved, I noticed I had sharp pain in my upper right arm and shoulder. When I looked to see what was causing the pain, I saw I had enormous bruising and swelling from where I had slammed against the granite countertop.

While I was in the hospital, physical therapists got me up and walking to build my strength. After three days, I was improved enough to go home. As I was being discharged, I was given a very thick report which contained all the information I would need to change my life. They said if I didn't want to have another stroke, all I had to do was read the report and follow the recommendations. I had already been told that the TIA was a warning. If I changed nothing, there was a good chance I would have other strokes, with each one more serious than the last. After this experience, I knew for sure I didn't want another stroke. I decided to follow every recommendation.

I'm a firm believer that it is never too late to do anything, or change anything and start over. I decided I had been given another chance to get it right and I better do my very best, or one of the next times I could lose my body altogether ... and it would be 100% my fault.

When I got home, I read my report, not only once, but several times and highlighted sections that I needed to remember clearly. At first it seemed more than I could possibly do. I already knew I had an addiction to food to soothe me for many reasons, over and above being hungry. I wondered, could I really quit this addiction? Food isn't like other forms of drugs that if you find the courage and determination to stop you live without it completely. Food is critical to survive. What I needed to be able to do was limit what I ate and how much. And setting limits on myself with food is something I had never been able to do before now.

My vitals were all there in the report, in black and white. My weight, 223 pounds, my BMI 42, and Obese level II. I didn't think I really looked obese. I always wore nice clothes that flattered me, or was I just living in denial about that as well? For once, I recognized that no matter what, these numbers were all dangerous statistics. I knew that if I didn't change, it was very likely I would have another stroke or a heart attack. I knew I had to do something, but where did I start?

My daughter Rebecca called me, "Mom, I'm worried about you trying to make this change in food all by yourself. I want to come over (she lives in MD/DC area) and help you clear out the pantry and restock everything with what you need to start over."

Rebecca and her husband both work full time and they have a small child. I hesitated before responding. "Rebecca, I'm happy you want to help, but I don't think it's a good idea to travel with Noah by yourself, or leave him behind with Jason, for you to help me right now. Plus, I think this is something I need to do for myself to really understand all the changes I am making and why. Why don't you wait, let me get started, we can compare notes with how I'm doing and you can give me suggestions over the phone or via email as I start making the changes?"

"Okay, Mom. But I just want you to know I want to help in any way I can. I don't want anything to happen to you. I want you to be around for a long time."

Rebecca did help by supporting me throughout my whole recovery process. She suggested new organic products for me to try, especially plant based butter, shared her favorite vegan recipes and websites with me and called me several times a week to check on me ... and to let my lovely grandson Noah tell me enthusiastically ... "Hello Grammy!"

With needing medication for high blood pressure and high cholesterol for years, going to no salt and low fat were the highest recommendations. I think I was most worried about giving up salt. I had been a salt addict all my life ... even adding it to McDonald's French Fries! But I also knew I had to overcome my addictions if I wanted to avoid another stroke. So I began. The first step was to clear my pantry and refrigerator of all foods high in sodium, fat and caffeine.

The hospital report gave me lots of recommendations and suggestions about what to eat and how much. But since I had never counted calories in my life, it proved to be a major lifestyle change for me. I was not embarking on a diet for a set amount of time to lose weight , but a dietary change that I would have to maintain the rest of my life if I wanted to live and have the full use of my body.

I made a promise to myself that I would do this. I wanted to live and I wanted to be active for as long as possible. The only way that was going to happen was if I learned all I could about nutrition and put it into effect in my life on a daily basis.

But the biggest promise I made was to my body. While looking into the mirror, I promised my body that from that day forward I would love, honor and cherish my body. And then I began talking to my body and touching each part of my body. I was so overcome with emotion that I was crying as I asked my body to forgive me. I needed forgiveness for neglecting, abusing and not ever listening to my body in my entire life.

And I reiterated my promise. I promised to listen, I promised to be conscious and choose what I put into my body so that everything coming in would be nutritious and helpful for my body to operate at the optimum level. And I promised to stop overeating so that my body didn't have to work so hard to undo the damage of what I put into it.

It was a powerful connection. I could feel the forgiveness wash over me. It was not too late. I could make amends by changing what and how much I ate. Now my body and I could go forward as true partners in life.

That was the beginning of me loving my body. I have kept my promise to my body and my body has become healthier and healthier since then. However, that is why the cancer diagnosis a year later was such a shock to me. *Why now? I got the lesson about taking care of my body and loving it when I had the stroke. Why do I need cancer, too?* It was later I learned that the cancer was there before the stroke happened. But no matter what, I still wondered what else I would need to learn from this experience.

Since having the transformation with my body and beginning to view it as my partner, my reaction to the cancer diagnosis was quite different than it might have been before. I didn't blame my body; I knew the cancer was not my body's fault. I felt compassion for it about the pain and discomfort it would go through during chemotherapy. Again, I talked to my body to prepare it for what was coming, and apologized that my body had to go through this at all.

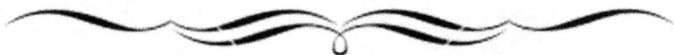

I believe I am responsible for the wellbeing of my body.

My body is my partner for life.

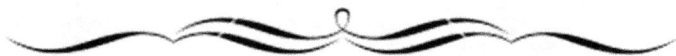

Chapter 12

Nutrition, Hydration & Exercise

I know that the chemo drugs are the first line of defense to kill the cancer cells in my body, but chemotherapy in and of itself can be hurtful to my body by killing some fast growing healthy cells in the process. I can't rely on chemotherapy alone to keep me healthy while going through this treatment. It is my responsibility to do everything within my power to keep my body healthy.

In researching ways to help myself stay healthier and minimize side effects of chemotherapy treatment, I learn that maintaining optimal nutrition, hydration and exercise in my daily life will help my body minimize the negative impact of chemotherapy. These three elements are the very foundation to live in excellent health before, during and after chemotherapy.

I have already promised my body I will do everything I can to help, but I wonder how I can keep everything up if I am not feeling well while in treatment. So, I make a plan to minimize the amount of effort that will be needed immediately following each chemo infusion treatment.

Nutrition

Fresh fruits and vegetables are the most important for me to have every day, so prior to a chemotherapy treatment, I stock the refrigerator so I have everything ready. I make a huge pot of vegetable lentil soup and freeze it in two cup portions so that it can be ready to eat with minimal preparation later.

For salads, I buy fresh organic baby spinach, green leaf lettuce, romaine lettuce, grape tomatoes, red onion, red pepper, cucumber and cauliflower.

For my vegetable lentil soup I buy celery, carrots, baby spinach, onions, garlic, red, green, orange, yellow and poblano peppers, lentils, unsalted vegetable stock, natural no salt added tomato paste and no salt added diced tomatoes with basil, garlic and oregano seasonings added.

For fruits I buy a combination of apples, grapes, bananas, melon (when fresh and available) and either blueberries or strawberries. Berries are extremely nutritious and a proven cancer fighting food. I was thrilled to learn grapes are considered a berry as big, crisp, juicy grapes are one of my favorite fruits.

I buy hummus to have for wraps and snacks, and sometimes I buy a low sodium whole chicken to bake and have for sandwiches. I eat a maximum of four eggs each week, and I buy fresh, organic brown eggs from cage free chickens. Even though I have not eliminated any food groups during this change, I do limit my meat and dairy consumption to the recommended guidelines. I switched to 1% milk and use it sparingly, I use low fat yogurt, a plant based butter and I only eat chicken, turkey and fish. I don't add sugar or salt to any food, and I have switched from white bread, a lifetime favorite, to wheat bread. In my desire to work toward more whole foods, I even begin baking my own wheat bread!

In addition to stocking my fresh fruits and vegetables and special items to make my soups, I check the pantry to make sure I have low sodium salad dressings, low sodium peanut butter, brown rice, low sodium crackers, saltine crackers with unsalted tops, low sodium pasta sauce, baking potatoes, sweet potatoes, walnuts, almonds, dried cranberries, oat bran, multi grain, oatmeal and wheat bread.

Now that I no longer use salt, I have researched and found many seasonings to help me overcome my addiction to having salt on my food. Mrs. Dash has a complete line of seasonings for multiple uses, all salt free. I use the original type frequently and the chicken or southwest chipotle seasoning for my ground turkey. I have the entire range in my pantry now.

Not cooking with salt was pretty difficult at first, but I have learned to compensate with new seasonings that are salt free. I never knew how many possible seasoning combinations there were! I like spicy foods, so those seasonings help compensate for not using any salt. Some I like to add to my vegetable lentil soup in addition to the original Mrs. Dash are cumin, tumeric, thyme, garlic powder, rosemary, parsley, cilantro, chili powder, red pepper flakes, cracked black pepper; to my salmon, dill weed and cracked black pepper, and to my chicken and turkey, Mrs. Dash and cracked black pepper. Hopefully I will always be able to use cracked black pepper when I cook, as it has become a major staple for me since I am not using salt.

I began eating healthily a year prior to my cancer diagnosis, and for that I am extremely grateful. At that time I cleared my pantry and refrigerator of all high fat and high sodium foods. I had a lot to throw away, and I did it without regret. And before my cancer diagnosis my change in eating habits had already produced concrete results. I was able to get off blood pressure medicine for the first time in decades!! And even during chemotherapy, with the exception of a few stress related blips on chemo days, I have been able to maintain normal blood pressure. Quite a miracle for me actually, the person who could never limit what she ate or when or how much before last year.

I've learned a lot about food in this past year. Of course I was somewhat obsessed in learning everything possible to help me to grow into excellent health. What I accomplished, I basically did on my own. Oh, I researched of course, and the hospital gave me a list of suggestions, but my accomplishments were in the spirit of healing my body, being kind to my body, loving my body, and helping it grow into excellent health that could last a lifetime without any damage to my body.

It was a slow process. I might compare my process to the race with the turtle who won the race by being slow and steady. I didn't want my body to be in shock from the changes. I didn't want my body to be in shock by any fast weight losses. I didn't want my body to have cravings for any specific foods simply because I eliminated an entire food group.

I took no diet pills. I took no supplements that were sold everywhere for weight loss. I didn't eat food prepared by anyone else. And I eliminated packaged foods, fast food, junk food, soda, caffeine, added sugar, added salt, high fat foods and high sodium foods.

I became a label reader, especially to confirm low sodium products. I was misled a few times by products labeled "low sodium" or "reduced sodium" on the front of the product when I didn't look at the ingredient label for the exact sodium content per serving. Although the label was correct, with the product being lower in sodium than their normal product, that didn't necessarily make it low enough for me.

Now, the only way I know for sure is to check the actual ingredient label. It is definitely worth it. I look for products with no more than 150 mg of sodium per serving. Plus I find out all the nutrients and serving size when reading the back label. There is way more information than just the total calorie count or sodium per serving. The ingredient label lists calories of fat from total calories, fat, sodium, carbohydrates, sugars, cholesterol, fiber, protein and potassium, serving size and of course, total calories. In watching food intake on a daily basis, and wanting to build and maintain a healthy body, each of these nutrients are important.

Although I didn't eliminate any food group, I was conscious of the recommended limits and stayed well within those.

Fortunately I'm not allergic to any foods, or diabetic, so I didn't have those concerns in limiting what I looked for in different ingredients on the labels. Even though I'm not diabetic, I'm still mindful of added sugar. And while I didn't limit carbohydrates as a quick way to lose weight, I continue to stay under the recommended limit of carbohydrates per day.

My main limits involve salt because of years of high blood pressure and needing medication to control it. Since I have eliminated salt as an add on, and only buy no salt added or unsalted products as ingredients for cooking, my blood pressure has become so regular and normal I no longer need blood pressure medication after taking it for many years.

Even products that offer no cholesterol, fat or sodium can vary brand to brand. So, even though I may find what works for me, I continue looking to make sure I am getting the absolute most in nutrition for every calorie I consume. I look at everything I eat from two standpoints. *Is this good for my body? Am I getting the optimal nutrition per calorie of what I am about to eat?* If I can have satisfactory answers to these questions, then I know I have the best possible food for myself.

One good example is my breakfast food. Before, when I ate oatmeal, I used the instant kind. I finally graduated up to the old fashioned oatmeal, but then I realized I get way more fiber and protein from oat bran hot cereal. So now that is my first choice for breakfast. Oat bran is the closest to the original oat and that is the best way to eat any product, as close to the natural state as possible.

My favorite way to prepare oat bran is adding cinnamon, a non-sugar sweetener plus chopped apple. Sometimes I have it with walnuts and dried cranberries or blueberries instead of the apple. Those just add a few more calories.

When I allow myself to have scrambled eggs for breakfast, I even make them healthier by adding a big handful of baby spinach and sliced grape tomatoes. Makes a beautiful plate, delicious and oh so healthy.

I find that many of the foods I am eating every day are considered super foods, especially spinach. And I eat a lot of organic baby spinach every day. I have a cup of baby spinach in my daily salad along with romaine and green leaf lettuce, I add six to eight cups of baby spinach when I cook my vegetable lentil soup, I use spinach in my wraps and I add fresh spinach to my scrambled eggs.

When I started eating healthily, with mostly fruits and vegetables, I already had cancer in my body ... I just didn't know it yet. I know that continuing to eat these super foods every day, especially after the cancer is gone from my body, will help me keep my body healthy and cancer free. And I think eating them while going through treatment will help the chemotherapy drugs do the best possible job for me in the process.

I do allow myself to have desserts as well. I just limit what I choose to eat and how much. Some things I have discovered as satisfying, and low in calorie impact, are angel food cake, fresh fruit, fat free whipped topping, cook and serve pudding made with 1% milk, ginger snap cookies, granola bars, no sugar added fruit popsicles and sugar free gelatin. The sugar free gelatin with the fat free whipped topping and fresh fruit on top is not only delicious, but low in caloric content and nutritious with the added fruit.

Although I didn't take any supplements to help me lose weight, which I think are not sustainable for a true permanent lifestyle change, I do take vitamins to help my body without tricking it. I take a multi vitamin, vitamin D, vitamin B12, calcium citrate, fish oil and fiber.

I was able to eliminate my blood pressure medication due to my lifestyle change. My hope for the future is that with my permanent lifestyle change I'll be able to clear my arteries so completely that the statin I have taken for years will no longer be necessary either.

Because of my lifetime of poor eating habits, high cholesterol for years and the stroke just last year, I think clearing my arteries will take more time for me to achieve. But I will keep eating healthily and never give up on this goal. I know that eventually I will achieve it.

Hydration

Drinking enough fluid is essential to help the chemotherapy drugs to work and flow through my body. Plus hydrating well helps to offset the drying effect the drugs have on the skin. After my first chemo treatment I was quite sick and could barely get any fluid into my body. I think not being able to keep myself hydrated in the beginning made it even more difficult for me to process the treatment. Since then I have become better and better about making sure I get enough fluid in my body every day, and now I am having almost no side effects from the chemotherapy treatments.

Because I no longer drink caffeinated beverages, I don't have to drink more fluid to make up for the dehydrating effect of consuming them. Ideally, water is the best possible liquid to drink, but I find it difficult to consume as much fluid as I need with plain water. I just don't care for the taste without some flavoring added. I found a great substitute in drinking Crystal Light, a powdered non-caffeine, non-carbonated and non-sugar drink, that is mixed with water. I can easily reach the minimum water goal of 64 ounces and most days reach my daily goal of 100 ounces. There are many different flavors of Crystal Light, and it's available in generic brands as well. My favorite flavor is raspberry lemonade. I know now that the more I drink, the better I feel.

I never leave the house without my container of raspberry lemonade and my "go to" food. Without either I face temptation for fast food and soda drinks while I am away from the house.

Exercise

Exercise is another critical element to healing while undergoing treatment for cancer. Anything helps. Moving my body helps. Prior to having my stroke I led a pretty sedentary life. Since then I walk approximately a mile every morning which gets my body moving and oxygenized. I also use free weights several days a week. I do my exercise lovingly and never push my body beyond its limits. Less than a year ago I was having so much pain in my back and left hip that I couldn't even walk to the corner. Now, I walk a mile every morning with very little effort or pain.

I am using every possible tool at my disposal to lovingly help my body go through cancer treatment. I want this treatment to be successful. I want to be totally healed when this treatment plan is completed. I am meditating, visualizing, writing, affirming, eating healthily, keeping myself hydrated and exercising every day. I am my own body's loving advocate during this chemotherapy treatment.

Chapter 13

Music, Meditation & Writing

As good nutrition, hydration and exercise are the three fundamental elements for me to build and maintain a healthy body, music, meditation and writing are my three fundamental elements to maintain a clean and healthy mind and spirit.

Since music can change my mood, I limit listening to soothing music that I can use in meditation and music that is uplifting. Music can tap into my emotions that are just below the surface and need to come forward for processing. Sometimes I'm not even aware I have something unresolved waiting to come forth until the music starts and I begin to meditate. And then, there it is. The best thing I can do is allow it to be expressed, regardless of what it is. Once it is expressed, then I am calm and can continue to meditate.

For me, meditation is very simple. I know there are all sorts of techniques for meditating, but I think that intent is all that really matters. The intent to go within and listen for whatever messages come forth. I do need a quiet place and to take time out, but only to be conscious and focus on my breath. The watching of my breath going in and out helps focus my mind. When I get distracted, and I do a lot since my mind is a very busy one, I just come back to focusing on my breath.

Saying a mantra, a phrase that I can repeat every time at the beginning of meditation, also can be helpful to go deeply into meditation. It isn't necessary, but again, it is something to help me focus. I choose to say *The Lord's Prayer,* usually a few times, when I first begin meditating. It reminds me of the spiritual power of meditation and prayer.

Although I do not list prayer as a separate fundamental element, my meditation experience becomes my prayer. In the silence I become present and receptive for God to guide me.

Writing is my therapy. The first thing every day I write. I get up very early, while it is still dark outside. I prepare a small pot of decaf coffee and I write in my office on my laptop computer without ever turning on any lights. My keyboard skills are very strong, and I can type much faster than I can write longhand.

I didn't grow up keeping a diary or writing journals, so I don't have that built in desire to feel my hands on the paper as I write. I'm much more comfortable using the computer. And I like writing in the dark with the only light being the light from the computer screen. It feels very intimate and enchanting. I don't put any limits on how much or how long I write. I write until I feel finished. I don't use prompts to write in the morning, but I always start and end the same. I start with gratitude. Gratitude for being alive, alert, in good health and writing. I have my two cups of decaf coffee while

I write, and my writing is always in the form of dialogue. As though I am having a conversation with a best friend, I write to God, or I could say my higher power. And I always end with "Bye for now ... we'll talk later ... Love you!"

I always ask for guidance, blessings and protection and I continually express my thanks and gratitude for what is happening in my life or with my family. And I write about whatever emotions I am experiencing. When I complete my writing, I am totally cleaned out of any unpleasant emotions, inspired and completely ready to start my day.

Right now I am keeping a daily cancer healing journal, a weight journal and I am writing this book. Writing is an incremental part of my life. It is healing, it is inspiring and I receive answers. As I write through problems, a resolution eventually presents itself.

This past year I was troubled because my husband was buried in our hometown nearly three hours away and it was not only inconvenient to visit him, I realized I did not want to be buried there. Oh, I wanted to be buried next to him, but I didn't want to be buried there. Plus, we had no money at the time he died and my sister paid for his funeral, his burial and the cemetery lots. It occurred to me if I were buried there, too, forever and throughout eternity I would be tied to her. And that is something I did not want.

But I didn't know what to do for sure. My logical mind told me it was impractical to make such a major change; that the cemetery lots were already paid for, and Jack was already buried there. *Was it so important that I should spend my savings to find cemetery lots here and then go through the expense of moving him?* When I talked to myself logically, I found myself thinking I should leave things as they had been for the past 40 years.

So I wrote about it. Over and over again I wrote about it. Finally I decided. I knew I did not want to be buried in the cemetery lots my sister paid for ... I wanted to be buried in Columbus, Ohio ... I wanted to move Jack ... and I wanted to buy lots for our children so that we could all be buried together. This was not a practical decision. It was more important. I was claiming my life as I wanted it to be, something I could not do at the time he died.

The timing of it all was incredible. The planning took months. I looked at 13 cemeteries. The longer I looked, the more discouraged I became. Columbus is a much larger city than Ironton, Ohio, and yet the beautiful Woodland Cemetery in Ironton seemed much nicer than anything I was finding in Columbus. And the cost for lots in some of the cemeteries was staggering to me. I began to have doubts I could pull this off.

And then I found Flint Cemetery, a small cemetery, co-managed by Sharon Township and the City of Worthington, Ohio. Located conveniently not very far from where I live, it was a very lovingly cared for, very quiet, serene and spiritual cemetery. They even had a meditation garden and a children's garden. I could breathe there. I could relax there. It felt more like a park than a cemetery. It was perfect.

From this point on it happened quickly. I learned that the moving of Jack must be done through a funeral director, and David Phillips of the Phillips Funeral Home in Ironton coordinated the move. He also made arrangements for one of his funeral directors to make the trip to Columbus, along with the vault company, just to make sure everything went smoothly in the move.

The Superintendant of Flint Cemetery had prepared the gravesite and awaited their arrival. My daughter Suzanne and I waited at the cemetery for their arrival as well. I came prepared with a big "Welcome Home" balloon for Jack as well as sage and incense to cleanse and bless the vault before it was lowered into the ground.

I had requested that the vault be power washed before leaving Ironton to remove the dirt from the last 40 years. As the vehicle transporting Jack's vault entered the cemetery and approached us, I literally gasped.

The company, Tri-State Wilbert Vault, had not only power washed the vault, they had painted it with a sparkling silver paint and it glistened in the sunlight! It looked even better than brand new. They had also tightly wrapped the vault in clear plastic so that no road dust got onto it during the transport. Their extra effort made me ecstatic, and I knew for sure I had made the right decision to move Jack.

I still used the sage to cleanse the gravesite and the entire vault as it was being lowered into the ground saying a prayer as I did it. I wanted to leave the pain of the past behind and celebrate Jack joining his family. And it seemed the tables had turned a bit. As long as Jack was alive, I followed him ... and this time, he followed me. In the past forty years, I have struggled, grown and built a wonderful life for myself and our family. And now it was possible for Jack to join us, at last.

His burial in this beautiful and serene cemetery was a major milestone. The timing was perfect as well. My goal was to have Jack moved no later than November 4th, the 40 year anniversary of his death. I met that goal for sure as the move was completed in late October. For the first time in these past 40 years I was able to spend the anniversary of his death, with him, at his gravesite.

For this milestone, I took incense and put one on his gravesite and took the other in a holder with me to the meditation garden. I could easily see his gravesite from there. As usual I started my meditation with *The Lord's Prayer,* and then asked for blessings for the cemetery and his gravesite. I was grateful to be able to enjoy this experience at last. Jack was finally home, with me and our family.

As I said, writing is therapy for me, and a major foundation element. Writing helps me heal ... express my gratitude and love ... resolve issues ... process feelings ... keep myself current ... and inspires me every day.

My commitment to daily writing is a direct result of the writing work I have done with Jeannetta Holliman. Her commitment to the importance of a daily writing practice, and expressing blessings while writing, resonated with me and gave me the framework that I use every morning now.

She recommends a 15 minute writing practice every day, but I don't limit my time. Jeannetta teaches that just starting ... even when it appears there is nothing to write about ... will bring something forth, and it is usually something important. Just keep writing Jeannetta says, no matter what, just keep writing. And I do. Every day.

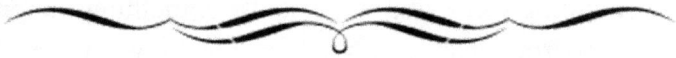

I believe that affirmations

can help us to become who we want

to be and to have what we want

in our lives.

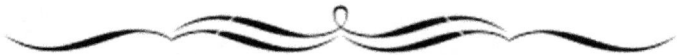

Chapter 14

Visualizations & Affirmations

Visualizations and affirmations are two powerful exercises that I use to help myself bring about positive changes I want in my life. My goal now is to remove this cancer from my body. Chemotherapy will do its part, but I don't think that alone is enough to ensure success.

I've been fully expecting to use visualizations and affirmations to help now, but lately, I haven't been able to get an image of the cancer lump under my eye shrinking. My daughter has asked me on more than one occasion, "Mom, are you visualizing the cancer tumor shrinking? You know that will help."

Every time she has asked me this question, I have mumbled an answer that I'm having difficulty seeing the tumor shrinking. I don't understand why I'm having difficulty. What is my problem? I'm feeling like a failure and a fraud that I can't do it. It doesn't seem real to me. Why not? I know in my heart of hearts it is real and I've never had any difficulty before, so why now?

I finally own up to Suzanne that something is wrong. For whatever reason, I'm unable to visualize shrinking the tumor. Nothing seems right. I'm feeling very badly about myself that I can't do something that I've done successfully many times before.

Then I read the report from the recent PET scan which describes the current status of the cancer under my left eye.

The cancer is in the muscle under my left eye! It is intertwined in the muscle and the muscle is quite enlarged. It is not a lump! No wonder I couldn't visualize shrinking a lump, the actual lump I had under my left lower eyelid is already gone!

I got it. I was trying to visualize the wrong thing. No wonder I couldn't see it. Once I had the right image, I could see it, and then I could see what to do to help it go away. I felt empowered again that I could help remove this cancer out of my body.

In meditation I visualized the muscle under my left eye and the cancer intertwined looking pretty much like the marbling on steak. Good image. I then asked that the cancer cells melt, floating through my body covered with Teflon, then out my waste being flushed away forever. I will do this every day while I am in treatment, until the cancer is completely gone.

And to back up this visualization, I write, print, sign, date and visibly post the following affirmation:

I Am Cancer Free

Now and

Forevermore!

Visualizations are images in the mind, best seen in meditation, and affirmations are expressed thought, in the present tense, preferably in writing, dated, signed and posted to be seen over and over again. The more reinforcement the visualizations and affirmations receive, the more powerful they are in bringing about the changes desired.

There are two other methods that can complement these tools; vision statements and dream boards. Vision statements, again written in present tense, are written for some future date. Usually five years or longer into the future.

While I was still working and in a meeting in Colorado with the Betsy Magness Leadership Institute group, our task was to write a vision statement for our lives five years in the future. Knowing I planned to retire in about five years, I went outside, sat at a table, meditated first, then began to write.

My vision statement wasn't long, but I wrote about the life I wanted and dreamed about for myself in retirement. It was written in great detail as though it was happening at that time, truly present tense. I could see my new home, including a large master bedroom and bath on the first floor and lovely wooded surroundings. All designed to fit my life and lifestyle in retirement perfectly. And every detail that I wrote about that day has come to pass, including living in my dream home, near my family and being a writer and author. Truly a powerful exercise to bring into reality whatever I can visualize.

A dream board is another way for me to affirm what I want to happen or have in my life. I use a poster board, then add pictures, images, or affirmations on the board. Then I post the board in a visible place where I can see it every day.

I had never travelled to Europe, and yet on one dream board I posted a picture of the Eiffel Tower. Within a year I travelled to Paris with my daughter Rebecca and actually saw the Eiffel Tower in person! It's time for me to make another dream board claiming that my cancer is totally and completely gone from my body.

It doesn't take much effort to work with visualizations or affirmations, and they go hand in hand. What I visualize can be reinforced with an affirmation. I write it, date it, sign it and post it. Each step helps to make the affirmation more real and helps to maintain focus on the goal to achieve the desired result. It does have to be written in present tense though. Words like I will, or I can are all future words and will keep the affirmation there, in the future. I bring the affirmation into the now by using "I am" in my statement as though it is already true.

Chapter 15

Dreams

Dreams also help me to tap into my subconscious. Although dreams are usually not literal, when one grabs me, and pulls me awake, I pay attention. I know this dream has a message of some type for me. I even believe in pre-cognitive dreams as well. I have had a few that helped prepare me for tragedy and dramatic changes in my life. Dreams that have a major impact as I awake are those I write down and date as soon as possible.

Unfortunately, my dreams fade pretty quickly after I wake and start my day. If I don't make note of it, in as much detail as I can remember, that dream or message is gone. I actually have a 3" binder notebook full of dreams I have written down and dated because they were significant enough in substance that I wanted to work on them for meaning and to remember them.

The pre-cognitive dreams are the most significant to me. These dreams I know are important when I have them but may not get confirmation of their connection to my reality until much later. I had two of these pre-cognitive dreams that literally told me of dramatic changes coming in my life. Because I paid attention to them, they helped prepare me.

The first dream with such an impact was when I was 34 years old, married with three young children and my husband was only weeks away from graduating from law school. It was to be his third advanced degree.

It was a Sunday afternoon nap when this dream came to me and I bolted awake in a deathly fear. In reality Jack was graduating from law school early, in December, and the plan was that he would start his law career right after graduation and I would remain in Columbus working until the school year was over. At that point I would sell our house and the children and I would move to wherever he had taken a job.

In the dream, all this took place. Jack had graduated, he had taken a job with a prestigious law firm in Miami, one of the places he was interviewing, and I stayed behind waiting for the school year to end before joining him. But in the dream, he never came back to get us. I waited and waited and waited, but he never came. I knew I was stuck in the house we bought to be temporary while he went to law school, and I was absolutely terrified. We had spent years on Jack building his education while I only had one year of college. Because of all the effort for his education we had no money saved, and there was no family to help. More importantly, Jack had always been my knight in shining armor and he was the holder of all our dreams.

When I awoke, I was hysterical and sobbing trying to tell Jack I didn't have any idea what I would do without him. He tried to soothe me by kissing my tears away saying nothing was going to happen ... but I had this nagging fear that would not leave me alone.

And then, just two weeks after I had this dream, Jack had interviews with law firms in Cincinnati, Ohio and he planned to spend the night. He didn't like to be away from me at night, but his happiness about our dreams being so close overshadowed his fear. He left early that morning, about 5 AM, and I was up with him. As we stood at the door, we hugged goodbye, and both of us had a hard time letting go. Finally he started out the door. I watched him drive away with both of us waving and smiling. He was out to capture our dreams.

That was the last moment I ever saw Jack alive. While in one of the interviews in Cincinnati, he started to not feel well, and left. While in his car driving, he suffered a massive heart attack and was dead before the ambulance reached him. My dream had been a warning. Jack had left to capture his dream, the job that would capture all our dreams, and he never came back to get us.

Jack's death was absolutely devastating to me, but I held onto my gratitude for the dream. In those last two weeks together, I was driven to spend every possible moment with him, making sure he knew how much I loved him. Because of the dream I was able to say goodbye to Jack, and live going forward without any regrets of our final days together.

The other pre-cognitive dream, that foretold a major life change for me, was actually predicting a positive change thank goodness. This dream occurred 14 years later than the one about Jack. And during these years I was very busy. When Jack died I was working as a secretary at United Cerebral Palsy of Columbus and Franklin County, and I didn't have the skills or education to grow beyond that position without major changes on my part.

Jack's sudden death changed the direction of my life forever. Fortunately for me, my new boss as of the morning he died, Gene Cuticchia, became the first and best mentor of my life. He supported as well as challenged me and taught me to look within for answers to my life. It worked. And change I did.

While working full time at UCP, I attended Franklin University one night a week for ten years and earned my degree in business administration. At the same time, my career at UCP had continued to advance until I was Director of Administration. And with Gene's support, while still working at UCP, I also started a consulting company working with other non-profits to help them prepare their budgets and accountability documentation for government funding. The name chosen for this venture was CBR & Associates, which represents not only my initials, but represents Cuticchia and Borromeo (our accountant and CPA) and of course Rosebrough.

Then, when I was 42 years old, I made a most important decision. After working at UCP for ten years, I left to take a job in cable television, a place where I could have the possibility of unlimited advancement and a retirement plan. As with UCP, my career advanced in cable as well. At the time I had this pre-cognitive dream, I was working as a general manager for one of the company's cable systems in Ohio.

This dream was somewhat coded as usual. I dreamed I was a state trooper, travelling with responsibilities between states. And the high top, lace up, dark brown leather boots that had been assigned to me were too big for me. In the dream, my first assignment was to an old, dark and dusty office with gray metal style furniture. As I travelled down a long hallway the next scene was an upgraded office environment with new furniture. Then I continued on and passed through double doors to be outside. It was sunny, the weather was perfect and I was on a grassy area by a beautiful cliff overlooking the ocean. Very peaceful, very scenic and wide open.

At the time I had this dream I knew it was important, but I couldn't quite figure out what it meant. The dream was in the spring, and in August I learned the cable system I managed in Ohio was to be merged with another and therefore my position would be eliminated. I didn't want to give up working for this company and lose what time I had toward vesting in my retirement plan, so I accepted a transfer to be the general manager of one of the company's cable systems in Pennsylvania. When I arrived there for the first time, I discovered the office building was old, dark and dusty with the gray metal furniture everywhere!

I still had a home in Ohio, so I truly was a state trooper driving back and forth for quite a while, until it seemed likely I would be in Pennsylvania long enough to purchase a home there. Not long after I assumed this position, I gutted the interior of this older office building, upgraded it, added all new furniture and created an inviting area for customers.

My career in Pennsylvania blossomed and my territory grew. Because of all my volunteering with local charitable organizations and using the company's television production as a resource for the community, excellent customer and government relations, and bringing out the best in the people working with me, I was recognized with awards at the local, state and national level including receiving the *Pennsylvania's Best 50 Women in Business* award from the governor of Pennsylvania. And best of all I was preparing myself financially for retirement.

The company that transferred me to Pennsylvania sold to another company, and they sold to another company and they sold to another company. In all these sales, I was retained as the general manager and even earned the title of vice president from the next to last company owning the cable system. By the time the last sale occurred, I was ready to retire and it was a good thing. The philosophy of this last company was to manage from either regional or corporate locations, and they didn't need a local general manager.

Because I was ready to retire when this last change in ownership happened, it turned out to be good news for me. I was 66 years of age, and had 24 consecutive years in the cable industry. Even though I worked for four different companies during this time, each successive new owner accepted my years of service from the prior company, and it was the same with this last owner. When my position was eliminated, they offered me a severance package encompassing all my 24 years of service even though I had only worked for this new company for 111 days!

The new company's decision to eliminate my position not only started my retirement, it let me live out the last part of my dream that I had years before. In the dream, the final scene was walking through double doors to a beautiful and scenic view that was wide open for me. In reality, I did walk through those doors, after retirement, by moving from Pennsylvania to Ohio to live near my children and grandchildren. I built a beautiful new home in Ohio on a lot with a scenic reserve of trees in the front and rear of my home. I am living the life of my dreams and life is wide open for me.

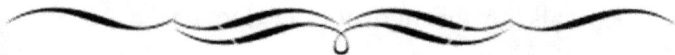

I believe there are no wrong turns,

only detours leading to

a new place of awareness.

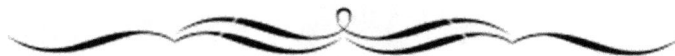

Chapter 16

Mid-Way PET Scan Results

Today I learn the results of my mid-way PET body scan and I am feeling some apprehension. Check-in is first, followed by my blood test in the lab, and a nurse checking my weight and vitals. At last it is time to meet with Dr. Patel.

He begins by asking if I have any questions and then moves to the scan report and hands me a copy. "Carol, the report confirms that your cancer has been reduced by 50%. We will continue with your present treatment for the last three chemotherapy treatments. However, even if the cancer is not completely gone after the sixth treatment, you will not have any further chemotherapy treatments. There will be another treatment at that time instead. We can talk more about that after we know the results when you are finished."

I am pleased that I have had a 50% improvement at the half-way point, but then I have a nagging thought that I recall Dr. Patel telling me he was looking for the cancer to be something less than that after this PET scan. Unfortunately this thought occurred to me after our meeting was over so I didn't have a chance to confirm it.

Today is my fourth chemotherapy treatment. When I arrive in the chemo infusion room, I learn I have a window seat assigned for me. Yeah! I love having a window seat because I have a wonderful view of the trees and I am not facing anyone else receiving a treatment. It gives me a little more privacy without being isolated.

I have come fully prepared for my day-long stay. I have three containers of Crystal Light, a humongous salad with all kinds of extras in small plastic bags that I can add at the last minute when I am ready to eat. I have freshly baked chicken, grape tomatoes, cucumbers, red peppers, cauliflower and shredded cheddar cheese to add to my romaine and green leaf and spinach. Healthy ... healthy ... and very healthy. I also have wheat crackers and red pepper hummus, half an apple, grapes and a low sodium peanut butter and jelly sandwich on wheat bread. No chance I will run out of food today and be tempted to eat anything not good for me!

As I get myself comfortable in the chair, the oncology nurse approaches me and confirms I have a port. Then I realize I did forget something today. I forgot to put Lidocaine cream on my port location to numb it before having the needle inserted for the IV. I am lucky. My nurse is quite skilled and the needle insertion into the port in my chest is basically painless ... even without the Lidocaine.

Now I'm ready to settle down for the day. I already have my jacket on, and then I put on my sleep mask and gloves and the nurse brings me a warm blanket. I tend to get cold during these treatments, but now that I know that, I come prepared. I already have my tape player ready with a guided meditation tape and turn it on. This is a tape I have listened to for over 25 years, and usually it is a wonderful experience.

Today is different somehow. The person speaking seems distracting rather than soothing. I quickly change to another one with music only, no words, and I naturally slip into a nice meditation. It isn't long before I am sound asleep.

I sleep now through most of the infusion period which actually makes the day go much faster. Today I notice a new person across the aisle off to my left side, and she has brought her own quilt with her. I love it. I presume someone has lovingly made this quilt for her, or with her. Perhaps her friends, or a church group made it, but it is a loving and beautiful way to be embraced while receiving chemotherapy. Each quilted piece has a message of hope, love or inspiration. It makes me think this woman must be greatly loved by a good many people for her to have been given such a gift. It gives me an idea for when I come for my next treatment. I will bring my own blanket. It won't have loving messages on it, but it will be mine and have my own loving energy in it. I am thankful for this woman giving me this idea.

This fourth treatment goes quickly and I am done even faster than ever. It is only 2:30 PM. It seems each treatment I am able to absorb the chemo a little faster and after four treatments I am finished at least two hours faster than the first treatment. Of course this means less traffic on the way home. Today has been a very good day.

My daughter Suzanne has been driving and accompanying me for all my chemotherapy trips to Zangmeister. In fact she has been a most wonderful friend to me, as always. She not only drives me and stays with me all day on chemo days, she also phones me several times a day on non chemo days to make sure I am doing well and whether or not I need anything.

It has been important for her to drive me on the day of chemo treatments. After all those chemicals going into my body for hours and hours, my body is in shock afterwards. I don't feel very stable to be on the highway driving myself home. But tomorrow I have my white blood cell booster shot scheduled at 3 PM and I will be driving myself. That is a very quick visit, only to get the shot, and I never have a reaction to it when I receive it. Because my chemo treatment is finished earlier today, it means that my appointment for my shot tomorrow is scheduled earlier in the day, too. It just has to be 24 hours after I finish the chemotherapy treatment.

I do drive myself for the Neulasta shot, and the trip is very uneventful. I leave early for the appointment, traffic is extremely light and I arrive quite early for my appointment. Fortunately I do not have to wait and I receive my shot, leave and am on my way home before my appointment time of 3 PM! Again, at this time of day, traffic is quite light and I am home without encountering any difficulties on the trip at all.

Following the fourth chemo infusion I think I'm ready to encounter any side effects that may occur. But I'm absolutely astounded! I have no side effects at all, except for the hyper activity from the steroid, Prednisone. I keep waiting for the side effects to happen, but they don't. I am prepared with everything I might need in the event I have side effects, but nothing emerges. It is fantastic!!

I wonder why. If the chemotherapy drugs have a cumulative effect on the body, why am I having such a good experience after the fourth treatment? I don't know. I'm confused, but I love it. I feel quite normal, and I'm enjoying feeling great immensely. I continue all my efforts to take care of myself during this time and I use this opportunity to make big batches of soup to freeze, to get some additional cleaning done in the house and to write, write, write.

I think I will ask Dr. Patel, when I go for my fifth chemotherapy treatment if the dosage of my treatment could be increased. It was reduced by 20% after the first treatment because of my side effects. If I'm no longer having side effects, it seems likely my chances of eliminating the cancer altogether would increase if the original dosage would be tried again. I only have two treatments left. If I can withstand whatever side effects I have on the fifth treatment from the increased dosage, then it could be used for both last treatments. And if I have serious side effects from the increased dosage, then the last treatment could be reduced again.

If increasing the dosage for these final treatments could possibly help me finish chemotherapy totally and completely cancer free, I am certainly willing to try it. Of course this is Dr. Patel's decision and he will have his reasons for whatever decision he makes. However, he always shares his opinion and the details of his decisions with me. And he is very willing to listen to my opinions and questions as well and incorporates what he can into my treatment. That I really like. I feel informed and a part of the process as I go through it. Now I can't wait until Monday to find out what he thinks of my idea.

Chapter 17

Co-Managing My Care

Today is my fifth and next to last scheduled chemotherapy treatment. Ever since I have been attending The Zangmeister Center for my cancer treatment, Dr. Patel has always been kind, patient and interested in my experiences with the treatment. When we meet, I know he already has a list of my calls with side effects since the last visit, but he still asks me to tell him what has happened since the last treatment. He listens with respect and then offers suggestions for me to try, or he alters the medication I am receiving to accommodate me. I never feel rushed or my concerns brushed aside. This environment of healing and cooperation validates and empowers me as I go through such uncertainty in healing this cancer.

Knowing that I plan to ask for my dosage to be increased on this visit back to the original level, I have prepared myself for possible side effects that could derail me from being self sufficient for a few days. Saturday and Sunday I cooked and shopped to purchase lots of fresh fruits and vegetables. Last week I had made another huge pot of my vegetable lentil soup with unsalted vegetable stock frozen into two cup containers. Very nutritious and delicious and can be prepared in a matter of minutes. My soup plus a large salad with green leaf, romaine and spinach and other nutritious toppings and I have a lunch prepared for a very heavenly, colorful and healthy lunch with practically no effort.

Saturday I cooked pureed asparagus soup ... another one of my favorites. It's very nutritious and delicious and contains nothing but asparagus, onions and unsalted chicken stock plus seasonings. Since I don't use salt, I find a little garlic powder, Mrs. Dash original seasoning (salt free of course) and cracked black pepper are all that I need to have delicious tasting asparagus soup with very low sodium.

On Sunday I baked a whole free range and organic chicken to have for sandwiches and salads. Although the free range organic chicken is more expensive, I find I can buy it at a reduced price on a manager's special when the sell by date is near. I don't mind because I know I can come straight home and bake it that day or the next. The other great thing about the free range is the additional meat I receive when it is deboned and the fact that no antibiotics are used. For me, those benefits make up for the incremental price difference. I have concluded the additional meat, especially on the thighs and legs must be the difference for the chickens, able to walk around rather than be caged.

To cook the chicken, I season it and wrap it tightly in aluminum foil to retain as much fluid as possible and bake it. Once the chicken is baked I remove the skin and bones, bag the chicken, date it and place it in the refrigerator. Again something nutritious, delicious and ready in minutes, or less, to use. I love having fresh chicken for sandwiches and salads. I haven't been able to use deli meat or packaged sandwich meat because the sodium count is way too high for me. Making my own, using a low sodium content chicken and baking it without salt, works perfectly. The free range organic chicken gives me that low sodium benefit with only 80 mg of sodium per serving. Most non-organic whole chickens usually have sodium content as much as three times higher.

It is 5 AM and I am up writing and preparing for my day of chemotherapy. Once I have completed my journal writing, I prepare my list of questions for Dr. Patel. I have a lot of questions, but of course the most important one is about increasing the dosage of my treatment today.

It is only mid-November, but we had a snow dump last night and it is still coming down. Plus it is below freezing. Normally I take my mile walk with my dog Buddy in the morning after I write, but it isn't safe for me to walk him in the dark with a heavy snow. Walking him will have to wait. It worries me because I am usually wiped out after a chemo treatment. Ever since I started with my chemotherapy I've been committed to exercising every day. So far I've never missed a day walking, not even on chemo treatment days. I wonder if it might be possible to walk Buddy after I get home.

As usual, my beloved daughter Suzanne is driving me to my chemo treatment today and for that I am extremely grateful. She calls to tell me that with the hazardous conditions this morning we need to leave early. Even schools are closing. I am already ready, my food and drinks are packed for the day, I have my sleep mask, my CD player, headphones and music, my gloves and for the first time ever I am taking my own blanket. But I won't have time for breakfast ... no problem, I have enough food for breakfast and lunch packed.

We make it to Zangmeister on time because we left early. Suzanne is quite a planner for arriving on time and she's a very cautious driver. Even though the traffic is bumper to bumper, heavy snow is falling and thick slushy snow is on the road, the entire trip is uneventful.

I am ready with my questions, all typed and I ask Suzanne to review my list. She has a few suggestions for additional questions and I just hand write those on my list so I don't forget anything. I even wore my beaded bracelet with the healing water from Our Lady of Lourdes today. I don't know why I haven't thought of wearing it before, but glad I did today. I think I will need all the heavenly assistance possible for my healing.

With the unexpected weather problems today, the center is running a bit behind. Normally they are like clockwork and I never have to wait for my appointment ... no problem. I just take the time to visit with my daughter and more questions emerge. I add them to my list, which has become quite long.

When I'm called for the appointment I learn I'm meeting with Dr. Patel's nurse practitioner today. My first reaction is panic. I've never met with anyone except Dr. Patel and I have all these questions. I can't imagine that the nurse practitioner can give me the answers.

When I question why I'm not meeting with Dr. Patel I learn that he normally rotates patients with his nurse practitioner and her name should have been on my schedule given at the end of my last chemo treatment. I hadn't noticed. I just made a note of the date and time of the appointment, expecting that Dr. Patel would meet with me. I check my schedule list, and there it is plain as day, my appointment is with Brittany Sweigart, not Dr. Patel.

With a little trepidation I express my concern to Brittany that I was expecting to meet with Dr. Patel and I have this long list of questions. Of course the biggest and most important one that can't wait is whether or not I can go back to the original dosage of chemotherapy on these last two scheduled visits.

She double checks the schedule and again tells me, no, there weren't any changes, my schedule was to meet with her. She even added that she was surprised she hadn't met with me yet because normally she and Dr. Patel rotate meeting with patients on every other visit. "Go ahead with your questions, I'll do my best to answer them, or get the answers for you."

I begin with the most important one. "During my last three week interval between treatments, I had no side effects at all. Now that I know what to do for all these side effects, I think I can handle going back to the original chemo dosage that I had on my first visit. Dr. Patel reduced it starting on my second visit by 20%. But since my cancer was only reduced by 50% at the half way mark, I think if the dosage is increased now my chances of having it completely gone at the end of chemo treatment is more likely. Mostly I would love to avoid having extended treatment after chemo is finished. I can't remember for sure, but I think Dr. Patel was hoping for something better than a 50% improvement at the half way mark."

Brittany asks me, "What side effects did you have that caused Dr. Patel to reduce your dosage?"

"Sores in my mouth, sore gums, sores on my lips, a few small spots on my face and a sore scalp. He told me he thought I would end up in the hospital if he didn't reduce it. Of course now I know what to do for myself if these return. I have my *Magic Mouthwash* which has kept my mouth and gums very healthy ever since then."

I'm delighted to hear Brittany say "I don't see any reason you can't go back to the original dosage. In looking at your records, he only reduced one drug, the Cyclophosphamide by 20% and of course he also reduced the Prednisone later from four tablets per day to three for the five day span. Also, did anyone tell you that you needed to have an IV iron treatment?"

"No, I haven't heard anything about needing an IV iron treatment."

Brittany then tells me that there are possible side effects from the iron, but that I am anemic and Dr. Patel added this treatment to my chart at my last visit. She also tells me that I'll receive this IV iron treatment on this visit and the next one.

My daughter asks her if I should be taking a supplemental iron at home in addition to the IV iron treatment I will receive today.

Brittany answers, "No, I think that the IV iron will work without adding anything at home. It's a dark brown liquid and as I said earlier, can have some side effects. It's best to wait to see what kind of reaction you have, if any, to the treatment today."

Some of my other questions were, "When will you test again to see if the cancer is all gone?"

Brittany tells me the testing will be done three weeks after my last treatment.

I then ask her about the 50% improvement I had in the cancer at my half way mark PET scan, wondering if it was expected to be more. I thought Dr. Patel was expecting a rating closer to three and I was only down to a seven.

Brittany explains a 50% improvement is certainly reasonable and one they see on a regular basis. She thinks this response reduction is pretty normal.

Flu shots weren't on the market yet this year when I started chemo and Dr. Patel didn't want me to get one after I started treatment. I ask her when I might be able to get one.

Brittany is surprised he asked me not to get a flu shot because he normally recommends patients get one. She tells me if I wait for two to three weeks after treatment is concluded that I should be fine to get one. But then she asks me "Do you know why he recommended you wait?"

"Yes, since I couldn't get one before starting chemo, he thought it would not be effective with the treatment I am getting, plus he also said I had a chance of actually getting the flu from the shot itself if I got it during treatment."

Then I ask Brittany ... "What will my treatment be, if by chance the cancer is not all gone when I have finished with chemotherapy?"

She says she can't answer that question and doubts whether Dr. Patel even knows the answer to that question at this stage. Since each patient is different and each treatment is tailored to the individual's need, she tells me he will wait until he sees the results and then what treatment would be best, if anything is needed at all.

"Next question ... I'm writing a memoir about my cancer healing experiences, and want it to be more of a documentary, including the chemotherapy treatment I am receiving at Zangmeister. I would like to use the center's name and Dr. Patel's name, but want to find out what protocol is necessary from Zangmeister before I publish. I would rather know before the book is finished so I can make adjustments if necessary."

"Well, Carol, you have stumped me. I thought I had heard every question there was to hear, and this is one I have never heard." She ponders a while, then responds, "I would contact the secretary to the President. Her name is Mary and she knows how to get everything done. Yes, I would start with her."

"Thank you so much, Brittany! You've been extremely helpful. Oh, by the way, I wanted to report some improvements I've noticed. The lump under my left eyelid seems to be completely gone. It's what alerted me to the problem that started the search for answers. Also the nasal drip that I've had since the surgery under my eye for the biopsy seems to have improved as well. Dr. Patel thought the drip was because of the loss of nasal hair, but now I think maybe it was from the lump under my eye pressing on my sinuses. If the tumor is shrinking it makes sense the nasal drip would be improving. And the double vision I was having is also completely gone now. I thought it was a result of the stroke I had, but now I think the double vision and the nasal drip were both caused by the cancer lump. I think these are all positive changes telling me the cancer is going away."

Brittany comes over and feels under my left lower eyelid where the lump was protruding. She thinks she can still feel a little swelling, but there is definitely no distinguishable lump as before. She compares it to the lower right eyelid area and she agrees, they seem pretty similar now. She thinks all of it is very good news and makes a note on my chart for the doctor.

This meeting has been great. All my questions were answered and now I have a contact person to ask about using Zangmeister's name in my book. Now onto my treatment upstairs in the infusion room.

I educate myself and make

responsible and informed

decisions.

Chapter 18

"Millie"

While waiting to be called for treatment, I realize I'm missing my bracelet. I literally panic. This is not a good sign that I've lost my bracelet that has been blessed and has a container of healing water. I look through all my things and can't find it. I remember getting my name band checked at the registration on the second floor so I check, but it's not there, nor is it downstairs.

When I get back to my chair in the waiting room I have a vague recollection I put my bracelet in an inside jacket pocket for safekeeping while I was getting vitals checked. Yeah! It is there! Now I can relax ... all is well.

My assigned seat today is not the row directly facing the window wall, but I do have a view of the windows and trees and no patient is seated directly across from me. It is perfect. I also have a new oncology nurse assigned today and she is extremely helpful. She is surprised I'm getting my lab work done downstairs with blood drawn through my arm veins before treatment when I have a port. I tell her that's how it's been done from the beginning. She says she'll put a note on the chart and schedule my blood work upstairs for the next chemo treatment so the port can be used. Then I'll go back downstairs to meet with the doctor prior to my treatment. It's pretty amazing actually. The drugs for my chemo infusion are not prepared until after I meet with my doctor. They are specific to me, and they are specific to what is needed each time. By waiting until after I meet with the doctor to prepare them, nothing is wasted and everything is freshly made according to what I need.

I like my chair today. It's different than the others, not terribly different, but somehow it supports my back a little better and it's easier for me to get out of by myself. I think this is going to be a very good treatment day. I get my bag of food and drinks set up on the left hand tray. The right hand tray is needed for the nurse to administer the treatment.

Today she explains that I will be getting the iron and gives me a handout of all the possible side effects. They sound pretty severe to me, but she adds that most people don't have a reaction at all. Then she asks if I need a drink to take my Tylenol with as I begin treatment.

I respond, "No, I have my own drinks," and I pull out my first container of Crystal Light.

When she asks if I want a warm blanket, I tell her "Thanks, I brought my own blanket today. I have everything I need for the day."

She smiles and says "I can see that. Just let me know if you do need anything."

Following that, the woman offering snacks and drinks comes by with her cart to see if I want anything.

Again, I respond. "Thank you, no. I have everything I need today." It feels so wonderful for me to be prepared for the day. I feel very well cared for by me. Now I understand why dreams I have had when I'm not prepared or can't find something I need panic me so. I like being prepared. Maybe it's because so much of my life I lived in a reactive mode, unprepared and bouncing from one crisis to another. I like being proactive about my life and my needs much better. I realize I have built myself a wonderful personal foundation and an automatic sprinkler system for my needs. This is a lesson I learned while in training to be a life coach and I love that I'm living it myself now, every day.

The treatment begins. I cover myself with my blanket, pull out my gloves, sleep mask, CD player and one of my favorite CDs. It is *Atlantis Angelis* by Patrick Bernhardt. As usual when the music begins I start my meditation with *The Lord's Prayer*. It has a calming effect, automatically taking me to a higher place. I become conscious of my breathing and breath. I am transported. The sleep mask blocks the overhead light, my gloves and blanket keep me toasty warm and the music blocks out any possible background noises or conversations. I totally relax and bless the drugs that are going through my body.

Although I've been having trouble getting visions about my healing, today is wonderful. I can see the drugs going through my body and I bless them to do their work and clear away this cancer. I also see a syringe type needle that is very thin but with a hole on the end that is sucking out all the microscopic cancer cells as the cancer drugs also enter the body. I love this vision! The cancer cells can be sucked up by the syringe and out to a waiting bag that can be disposed of through medical waste. So much better than my previous vision where they travelled through my body and out my waste. Cancer cells having to travel through my body means any stray cell breaking off could become rogue and start up the cancer somewhere else in my body!

The time passes quickly and my CD finishes. I'm still awake and start a new one. Another favorite called *Yoga Sound* by Wai Lana & Siddha. As soon as it begins, I start feeling emotional. There is nothing like certain music to evoke feelings hidden just below the surface.

And then I have the image of Millie sitting on my cheek. Millie is the name I have for my cancer. My daughter Suzanne had a vision of my cancer looking like a millipede wrapped tightly around my left eye muscle. She decided to ask the millipede to leave, but he responded by saying that I still needed him. He let go of my eye muscle and instead came to sit on my cheek, ready to go back in at any moment. At least this was a step in the right direction.

After Suzanne told me about her vision, I was angry and tried to force Millie to leave. But he would not budge. Suzanne had a later vision with Millie's head hanging low and looking quite sad. She asked what was wrong and he said he was sad because I was angry with him. He also said he didn't want to leave because he liked me and thought he was helping me.

With that news I began visualizing Millie, asking him what I still needed to learn. What message did Millie have for me? First I was told I needed to promise I would finish this book and to include a story about Millie and how he helped me. I agreed and I promised him I would do both.

For the first time since I received my diagnosis of cancer, I realized that I had never blessed the cancer and thanked it for giving me the lessons I still needed to learn. Millie wanted recognition for helping me, but now that job was over and it was time for him to leave. But how do I get him to leave voluntarily? He's definitely not leaving by force for sure.

When I realized he truly had accomplished his mission with me and only wanted recognition for his efforts, I thought of course. He needs a promotion. He has won his wings! And my daughter, Suzanne, with her expertise in chemistry, had already told me that matter cannot ever disappear, it just takes another form. With that in mind, I know I am doing the right thing imaging a promotion for Millie and acknowledging what a good job he has done for me.

So, as I am listening to *Yoga Sound* and nothing else exists for me outside my meditation, I see Millie sitting on my cheek. Wings and all. As I am saying thank you for his contributions, an angel, glowing and all in white, suddenly appears. Millie is ecstatic. She has come for him. I had no idea that even though he knew he was finished with his assignment for me, he was afraid to leave and be alone because he didn't know what to do or where to go. Total love exudes from this angel and she leans over to scoop up

Millie and he throws his arms around her neck. They fly away together.

And then I hear the message. "Your cancer is gone." A wave fills my body and flows through it with a whoosh, as though the cancer is rushing out to leave my body. Overwhelmed with emotion, I am crying and love literally overflows the bounds of my body. I know, at some highest level, that my cancer is gone. Just as I have been affirming over and over again.

And then I sleep. I don't even know when my music ends and I never remove the headphones. I sleep until it is nearly time for the treatment to be over. I awake refreshed without my body feeling in shock at all. It is unusual and for the first time I feel quite normal at the end of a treatment. What is odd is that I had an increased dosage of chemo drugs and the added iron. The healing I experienced must have been total, including helping the drugs go through my body totally unimpeded.

The drive home is wonderful. I feel great, the traffic is less, the roads are clear and we get home as early as the last time. Since I am feeling normal, I decide to take Buddy for his daily walk. I am so pleased with him. Even though he didn't get his walk this morning, he didn't mess in the house while I was gone all day for treatment.

I put the ice cleats on my shoes and dress myself and Buddy for the cold, ice and snow waiting for us outside. It is tough walking as there is a lot of ice on the sidewalks, but I am careful and I feel safe wearing my ice cleats. We walk our normal mile and I return home filled with gratitude, thanking God for all he has done for me and continues to do every day. I feel hopeful and inspired by the events of the day.

In keeping my promise to write about Millie, I hope that he is pleased with how I have recognized his contribution to me and that he is proud I have named a chapter after him.

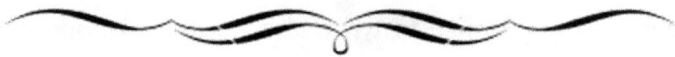

I believe in angels and the power

of the unseen world.

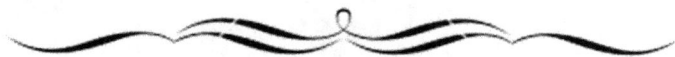

Chapter 19

After Care

By asking to have an increase in my cancer drug dosage yesterday, I fully expect that I will have side effect repercussions similar to after my first treatment. However, I am no longer a novice in my cancer treatment and have remedies to help myself for every side effect I have experienced so far. And I also know that in those first few days after treatment I am the most vulnerable for infections and side effects. I am ready to double up and take care of myself through every minute of every day.

While I still have some energy after treatment and walking Buddy, I have asparagus soup and my leftovers from Zangmeister for dinner. Then I unload the dishwasher that I had turned on before leaving this morning and clean up my containers and dishes. I put the blanket, my gloves and sleep mask that I had used during the day in the washer, and my clothes, towels, pajamas and my cloth CPAP liner in the laundry tub for the next wash.

Then I start getting ready for the evening. I take my evening meds and floss, use my two electric toothbrushes and my magic mouthwash. Even though my mouth is fine today, I know I need to be super diligent keeping my mouth clean and medicated to minimize any opportunity for the sores to return after having this increased chemo dosage. Next I shower, put body lotion on all over, use lip balm to keep my lips moist through the night, cocoa butter to keep my hands from drying out, put on clean pajamas and climb into my clean bed.

One of my favorite television shows is on PBS tonight at 9 PM. It will be a great reward for a great day to watch it. I manage to stay awake and watch the show, which is another terrific episode and coincidentally the final. So glad I didn't miss it. I don't have a television in my living room as I only watch it when I am in bed. I have a 50" flat screen television on my bedroom dresser so it is like watching a home theater from the comfort of my own king sized bed! Very enjoyable. So enjoyable in fact I truly have to limit how much, and what I watch, as I have a tendency to lose track of time. As much as I hate to admit it, television watching for me can be addictive and an escape. Before I know it I can fritter away hours while I watch mindlessly.

My only side effect the next day after treatment is the hyper energy from the Prednisone steroid. But, no other side effects, which is an absolute miracle. No nausea as after my first treatment. No flushing as after my second treatment. And nausea was one of the possible side effects from the addition of the iron. So, very good news having neither. Of course I have the anti nausea medication just in case. Better if I don't need it, but I am prepared if I do. No sores in my mouth yet, but those started a few days after treatment before. Hopefully I can keep those from happening, being proactive with my increased self care.

It is even colder today, 16 degrees, and the sidewalks are still covered with snow and ice. Some neighbors have been very thoughtful and cleared them right away, but not everyone has done that. It makes walking treacherous for me. I'm wearing my safety ice cleats. They help stabilize me on the ice and the balancing training I received from physical therapy also seems to be paying off. At 74 years of age, and having hurt myself seriously in falls before, I know a fall now would set me back big time.

I wear thermal underwear under my clothes and my normal hat, gloves, scarf wrapped around my face and my new packable down jacket which is supposed to keep me warm down to zero degrees. So far I have not been disappointed. Buddy has his heaviest jacket on, too, and we begin. He loves his daily walks and prances all around until we are on our way. We make it to the corner and turn to go up a street that has a tree reserve off to the side, but no houses and only small trees along the sidewalk. The wind is bitterly cold and fierce. I am okay, but Buddy is not. He is a rescued rat terrier and only weighs 18 pounds. His ears are pinned back from the wind and for the first time ever, he stops, turns around and looks at me. He can't take it and wants to go home! We turn around to head toward home, but once we get off this street, houses shield the wind and he is ready to continue on his walk after all. I am grateful that even under these conditions I am able to walk my mile with Buddy.

One of the wonderful benefits of my visits to Zangmeister is that I receive a copy of all the details of my visit, my vitals and the individual blood test results before I leave on chemo days. To keep track of my progress and changes, I created an Excel spreadsheet for each visit's results as well as the range of normalcy for each one. Today I included my results from yesterday on the chart and I noticed some changes that aren't good.

My white blood cell count has dropped to 5.56, my lowest so far. Fortunately that's still in the normal range of 4.4 - 11. I'm certain the Neulasta shot I get the day after every treatment to build white blood cell count in my bone marrow is helping to keep this in the normal range.

However, there are two changes that are worrisome. The red blood cell count is 3.72 and the normal range is 4.1 - 5.43 and the hemoglobin is 11.3 with the normal range 11.9 - 16. Both these categories have fallen below the normal range. Perhaps that is why the IV iron was added to my recent chemo infusion treatment. When I was told I was anemic, I didn't ask which category caused this conclusion. As I look at my spread sheet I notice these two were below normal at my previous chemo treatment as well.

My iron level is not listed on this particular report, but I located it on another one. No wonder they added iron during my treatments ... my iron has dropped nearly in half since I started chemo.

The other category that is still worrisome is the Immature Grans #. It is supposed to be at 0.00 and in the last two treatment results they are at 0.02, which doesn't sound like much of a difference. But I think it is the only indication that I might still have some cancer cells in my system. Mine started out in the beginning at only 0.01, not much of an indication that I had cancer. However, that number grew to be as high as 0.06 when I was tested at my second chemo treatment. It has gradually declined during treatment. These cells start out in the bone marrow and are supposed to mature into some other form of granulocyte before going out into the body. I suppose those that don't mature could escape to be rogue cells.

It's a good thing I was writing about my Neulasta shot today. The Prednisone pills I took this morning have had me in quite a hyper task mode all day and I totally forgot my appointment for the shot today at 3 PM! In looking at the computer clock it is already 2:10 PM. It's late, but not too late, I can still make it.

The steroid Prednisone has been part of my chemotherapy treatment from the beginning. I receive it on treatment day, in the IV in addition to the chemo drugs, and then I take it in pill form at home for the first five days after treatment. It helps to curb side effects from the chemo drugs, and I think helps to reduce the fatigue that I would experience without it.

I use the term hyper task mode loosely in how I describe my reaction. This is a term my children made up years ago to describe me when I am highly energized, motivated and driven to complete a task. And this is how I feel taking Prednisone. Literally being very busy and driven to complete tasks, to the point of my mind racing to what I need to do next, not really being able to fully relax or sleep for any length of time.

Even with my delay leaving for the Neulasta appointment today, I do make it on time. I'm registered and in my seat in the waiting area at 2:59 PM. The rushing stresses me out and the stress on my body shows up in my blood pressure. It is quite elevated when Kenya takes my vitals. It is 153 over 65. I think the 153 is my highest yet on any of my appointments at Zangmeister. Afterwards I wonder how much of the blood pressure elevation is from my stress or perhaps how much is due to my hyper task mode from my Prednisone prescription.

I decide to take my blood pressure this morning to check it for a comparison. I have already had my Prednisone pills so any influence they have should show up in the results. My blood pressure is quite low, 77 over 57 with a pulse of 78. I'm shocked to discover my blood pressure elevation yesterday was strictly from the stress. And I trust my blood pressure machine for reliability. It's my third one, because the first two I had were not reliable or consistent at all. It was very frustrating until I purchased this one which is an OMRON BP785 and I really like it.

Because I have had a history of high blood pressure for years and taking medication to lower it for years, I am quite sensitive to any changes in it. With having my own reliable blood pressure machine at home, I take my blood pressure regularly, and document the results on the computer, to make sure I am staying within range of normal.

With my dietary changes, weight loss and not eating any salt for over a year, I was able to get off blood pressure medication completely and have had no ongoing recurrence of high blood pressure since then, even without the medication. And that is a benefit I want to keep. I don't think I've ever been able to notice, for sure, that stress alone can elevate my blood pressure. Getting this confirmation today surely makes a great case for me to continue meditating every day to calm my body. There are many other benefits for me to meditate, but calming the blood pressure in my body is not one that I had claimed yet. I do so now.

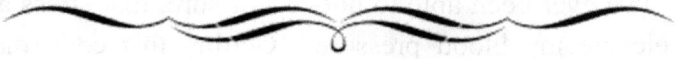

I believe that meditation and writing

are the paths within.

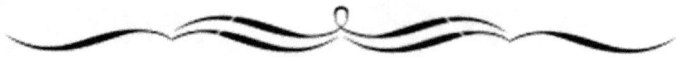

Chapter 20

Forgiveness

Forgiveness is the gateway to healing. And I think lack of forgiveness is the biggest block to healing and personal growth. Whenever I have not been able to forgive another, or myself, I am held in bondage to that event or person until I can release the attachment.

Of course forgiveness does not mean condoning or forgetting, it is strictly letting go of whatever I have not been able to forgive. And the process is actually very freeing. The Buddha teaches that the greatest suffering comes from attachment. This is very true in the case of not being able to forgive.

In my case, I suffered a lot of trauma at the hands of people who should have loved, cared for and protected me, but did not. There were lots of people and lots of events to forgive, in order for me to heal and become whole and free. It is possible. It takes time, it takes work but it does happen. Oddly enough I have found the hardest person to forgive is myself.

All of us have that inner voice that tries to guide us in our actions and decisions. Unfortunately unmet needs can sometimes scream louder and drown out this voice. Every single time I have betrayed myself, not listened to my inner voice and followed the screaming unmet need instead, it has been a wrong decision for me. Not that I didn't learn from it, I did every time, but in the meantime I delayed myself from fully living my own life.

Of course I also believe there are no accidents. Those decisions where I tried to fulfill unmet needs usually led me to what I really needed to learn and more directly within to myself.

But the times I betrayed myself, sometimes for lack of courage to say "no," were like poison inside me and festered until I could grow strong enough to truly look at what happened and to work through to forgiveness of myself. Why it's harder to forgive myself than another, I don't know. I just know that's the way it works for me.

As I write this, I think of Swami Shantanand "Shantji" Saraswati, a dear and loving friend I met nearly 25 years ago while working in Pennsylvania. Shantji was born, raised and educated in Allahabad, India. He still has an Ashram in Allahabad on the Ganges River and the cave he lived in for years, but now he lives primarily in his home and Shanti Temple in Montrose, Pennsylvania.

It was during the years Shantji was living in his cave that he honed his beliefs, purified himself and discovered what he calls the *Wisdom of Non Doing.* The premise being that we are not doers, but our history, internal mechanisms and thoughts drive us to the actions that we eventually take. As we grow and change we update these mechanisms and different parts gain strength which can lessen the struggle within when decisions are needed.

This teaching resonates with me because of the struggles I have had with decisions in the past and not understanding when some were made not in my best interest, but being drawn to make them regardless.

And most of all, Shantji's teaching helped me begin to fully accept myself during what Dr. Charles Whitfield, in his book, *Healing the Child Within* so aptly named for me, age regressions.

Without anyone to help me process the many wounds happening in my childhood, the memories and pain were buried in my unconscious. However, being buried in the unconscious doesn't mean they are gone.

Unfortunately, this process of calling forth emotions from a buried trauma cannot be done from an intellectual level. For me it only happens when a current event triggers a past trauma. The piercing of the memory capsule, hidden deep within, can be triggered by something small. A look, a sound, an energy that is similar enough to what happened in the past zaps through the years and the buried emotions of that long ago event rush forward. In that moment, when that happens, I become the age I was when the trauma occurred.

The first time I was aware enough to know something happened beyond what I could handle, it scared me greatly. I was at a weekend role playing workshop for interpersonal communication and the last role play was underway. I was just on the sidelines for this one. The scene was very intense, and I was unaware I had been holding my breath. As the participants made contact, I was so relieved I let out a sigh, which I think must have come out as a small laugh and it broke the concentration.

In that instant, everything stopped and it seemed everyone turned and glared at me ... I felt immediate shame as though they were all pointing their fingers at me and saying "Shame on you ... it's all your fault!" and blaming me for ruining everything.

All of a sudden, I became 14 years old at my mother's funeral when my cousin pointed her finger at me and accused me for being the reason my mother was dead. She had been the housekeeper for my mother while she was ill and she hated me with a passion. I was a sassy kid and I didn't want to help her with the housework, so she got more than even with me that day.

When this happened at the funeral I ran to the bathroom sobbing and I threw up over and over again until nothing was left inside me at all. I never told anyone what Cousin Nettie did to me, and this event and my sassiness became buried for decades.

The trigger at the role play brought forth all those unresolved feelings in a flash. Again, I ran to the bathroom, this time sobbing with dry heaves and I held onto the sink to keep from collapsing. I tried to stifle my crying, but it just wouldn't stop. It didn't take long for my face to become blood red and my eyes swollen. I was afraid to leave the bathroom in that condition. I kept throwing cold water on my face knowing eventually I needed to rejoin the group. Somehow I recognized my emotions from that day at the funeral, but had no idea what had just happened to me or why.

I did rejoin the group. But at that point I felt like an alien and definitely didn't belong. Everyone was happy, hugging each other and saying their goodbyes, while I felt like a zombie and quite invisible. If this had not been at the finale of the weekend, perhaps I might have had a chance to work through what happened with the facilitators, but it was over. No one even noticed me or that I was not okay. At that point my body was in so much shock I was unable to ask for help or take care of myself. While everyone else was busy, I picked up my things, totally bewildered by what had just happened and started home.

My first step in really understanding these regressions, and what to do for myself, came from Dr. Whitfield's book and description of the process of age regressions. After that, I discovered tools to help myself get through one as quickly as possible.

Most people have no understanding of these age regressions. When one happens to me, on the surface it appears I am just overreacting to nothing. Now I know better. I know to remove myself as quickly as possible from other people, get to a quiet place where I can bring myself back to the current time, settle myself, understand what has happened and why, and then I can return with other people. The exception to this is with my daughter Suzanne, who also understands this process and is my best resource if I ever need help processing through one.

Fortunately, with years of therapy and years of experience working through the emotions brought forth by these memory capsule piercings ... and *lots and lots* of forgiveness, I can honestly say they rarely happen to me anymore. However, at this point if I have a big reaction to an event or another person, that is disproportionate to current reality, it is pretty certain I have had a memory piercing of a long ago unresolved trauma.

After meeting Shantji, and hearing of his philosophy of the *Wisdom of Non Doing*, I have come to accept these age regressions as part of me and nothing I can control. In the past, especially when I first became aware of them, I tried to stop them. Or I felt shame that I was not able to control my emotions. Once I accepted these as normal, for me, the real healing and forgiveness of myself began.

Now if I have an age regression, it still isn't easy, but I understand it and accept it. I know that if I can just stay with the emotions coming forth, I will eventually return to the present time with something very important healed within me.

To me this experience feels similar to falling into a void or deep hole. Feelings triggered are usually fear, confusion and shame. Very much a sense of not being in control and not tethered to anything. Sounds scary, doesn't it? And without any understanding of what is happening, it is scary. However, l have finally come to trust that these events always lead to my greater healing, understanding and my highest good.

Several weeks after I started chemotherapy, an email from an old high school friend informed me that my brother-in-law had died and she was writing to express her condolences. She mentioned what a great guy she thought he was. I had to smile. He truly did have a great public face, was a deacon in his church and prayed on his knees every night ... right after he molested me!

My daughter later found his glowing obituary on the Internet and the date of his death was ... the very day *before* I started chemotherapy!

Of all the people in my life I needed to forgive, he was the hardest and took the longest because the damage that occurred lived within me most of my life. And even though I had forgiven him, I no longer wanted him in my life in any way. As I said earlier, forgiveness does not mean condoning or forgetting, it is just a process to let go of the past, the wounds and heal the wounded spirit.

The timing of his death seemed almost miraculous to me. Chemotherapy drugs were going through my body to kill cancer cells starting the day after he died! I imagined now that the chemo drugs were also erasing any last traces there might still be inside me from my brother-in-law's actions all those years ago when I was just a teenager. I now know for sure that I am coming through this cancer healing process clean and healed in all ways!

I will forever be grateful to Dr. Charles Whitfield for writing about, describing and naming age regressions for me in his *Healing the Child Within* book. And for Shantji, through his *Wisdom of Non Doing,* for giving me a way to accept them plus trust myself while in the midst of one.

Because forgiveness is so key for me to heal and move forward with my life, I have a ritual I use whenever I feel a need to forgive myself or someone else. It is very simple, and yet quite profound.

I meditate first to center myself. Then I write a letter to the person I want to release from me. I don't worry about anyone ever reading what I write because once I have finished processing everything possible, I burn the letter.

I write through every feeling and emotion that comes forth, regardless of anger, guilt, blame, rage, fear or shame, etc. I no longer fear the emotions coming forth thinking they are too much for me to process. Staying with the emotions, honoring and writing through them is the best way for them to eventually pass or subside. I have had times with this exercise when my energy was so strong that my pen actually tore the paper. Since I do this exercise when I'm alone, I can scream bloody murder when I need or want to do so. Sometimes it takes a while for the emotions to emerge, but if I'm patient and continue to write, the emotions will surface.

When I have nothing left to write, I'm ready to burn the letter. Sometimes I'm exhausted and can have several pages, depending on what has come forth. There is no right way or right number of pages. The right way is as it happens. The whole process is just to release the poisoned memories out of me.

When I'm ready to burn the letter, I fold it lengthwise and tear it in half. Then I fold each half in about three folds. With each half page loosely held at the corner, it makes it easier to burn. I also prepare a large bowl of water and of course I need a match or lighter. As I burn each half sheet, I hold the burning paper over the bowl and repeat three times that all is forgiven between us, (and this works the same as when I am forgiving myself) that both of us are released and free now and forevermore. When I am completed burning all the pages, I pour the water and the ashes into the toilet and flush all of it down the drain. As in the case with my brother-in-law, I needed to do this exercise many times. I have learned that this ritual eventually gives me freedom from whomever or whatever has held me in bondage.

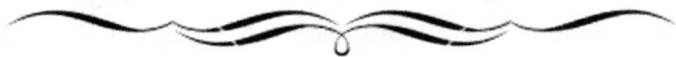

I believe that forgiveness is

the gateway to healing.

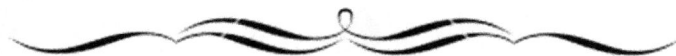

Chapter 21

The Art of Being Deliberate

Growing up as I did, I was never introspective, reflective or inner directed. All my energy went to being on hyper alert watching those around me for what might be coming next. I became an expert at reading another's mood through their energy or facial or bodily expressions and how to stay out of their way to avoid conflict. It took years for me to begin an inward journey and to shift my focus there instead of feeling a need to protect myself from others.

The change did happen though, little by little, baby steps even. One of the lessons I have gained, going through chemotherapy treatment, is that I have finally arrived at a stage in my life that I can claim the art of being deliberate. It sounds simple enough, but it is not so simple.

To me the art of being deliberate is to be mindful of my thoughts, decisions and actions as much of every day as possible. This shift in my thinking, conscious behavior and ability to live deliberately is very important. Otherwise I can drift aimlessly through life and let valuable time fritter away. The only exception to my living deliberately now is when I have an age regression and go on auto pilot with unconscious behavior. Fortunately these rarely occur anymore.

For 34 years I worked for other people. I was the sole support of myself and my family after Jack died. Beginning without a solid financial, educational or emotional foundation I lived in fear that someone could fire me and there would be no one to step in to help. So, my workaholic self was born in terror during these times. As my career soared, that fear lessened over time, but in fact I never completely lost it. The important piece is that during these 34 years I worked and lived on someone else's schedule.

While I was still working, I graduated from Coach University as a life coach and I also became a certified retirement coach through Retirement Options. The training in both was extremely helpful to me personally.

As I was in the process of retiring and completed my own retirement readiness assessment with Retirement Options, the results were that I was very identified with my job. That made sense because I had a great deal of joy in my work, was very successful and received lots of praise and recognition for my efforts.

When I retired, my life had no schedule. I didn't need to be anywhere, anytime, or meet with anyone. There were no expectations of me other than those I had of myself. The combination of shifting from a lifetime of being on someone else's schedule to none, and my identity with a job where I received lots of positive feedback to none in retirement was quite a shock. Of course I was overjoyed to not have the responsibility of working, not living on someone else's schedule or needing to do corporate budgets any longer.

But it never occurred to me that if I didn't have any schedule at all, there was a great possibility of me wasting valuable time. And now, at 74 years of age, time for me is becoming more and more of a limited commodity.

Because of those 34 years of living on other people's schedules, at first I was adamant I wanted no schedule when I retired. Over time it became clear that my stubbornness about not having a schedule was not such a good idea. Gradually I saw myself drifting into watching more television and getting caught up in other people's worlds rather than fully living mine. And during this time I was still unconscious of my body and ate terribly. I was still quite childlike in what I wanted to eat and didn't really want the trouble of cooking for myself.

One good thing that happened in this life change was my commitment to writing. I found writing helped me find my own voice and decide what I wanted for myself in my new life. I began eliminating everything toxic from my life or anything that I had just been tolerating before. I finally began setting limits on myself and on others. I realized that my difficulties in setting limits on others had to start with me. I didn't want to accept the word "no" from myself when I wanted something. I found I had quite the rebel inside who balked when she wanted something.

This lack of setting limits, this internal rebel, affected how I spent my time and how I ate. I have learned a technique for my rebel which works for the first time in my life. Instead of an outright "no" to eating too much, I ask her if she can wait a little while, and I give her the time when she can eat. Since

I have changed how, what and when I eat, I like to let at least three hours go by between meals. I think this time gives my body a chance to digest what I have just eaten and gives me an opportunity to at least get a little hungry before eating again. However, my shift to eating nutritious food has been extremely calming for my body and my internal rebel. This has been a wonderful revelation to me.

When I was overeating all the time, it was never because of real hunger. I don't think I ever let myself get hungry. I ate for a zillion other reasons ... anxiety seemed to be the major culprit. Especially the floating anxiety when I didn't know the real cause. In the past food always sedated me in those situations. Now I use other ways to soothe myself. And writing is a big one. I write through my anxiety and usually find the cause. Once I have the cause, I can write and work through the feelings associated with the cause and usually resolve the problem while writing. Meditation is my other resource to calm myself plus receive answers to my concerns.

However, it was the TIA warning stroke that I had in August a year ago that was my wakeup call about taking care of my body. That was a major step leading me to this final stage of being able to live at a deliberate level in all areas of my life. I now know that I am fully responsible and in charge of my life, my time, my body, my health, my spirit, my money and my happiness ... no one else. It is an empowering thought and fills me with such gratitude to arrive at such a wonderful place in my life. Taking full responsibility for myself and all areas of my life has given me my freedom ... a lifelong dream. I am content.

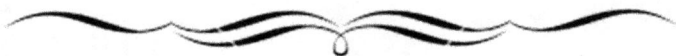

I am responsible and practice

the art of being deliberate daily.

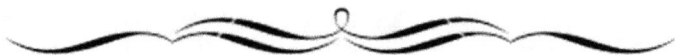

Chapter 22

Fifth Treatment Side Effects

Miracle of all miracles, I'm not having any of the serious side effects I was expecting to have with the increase in the chemotherapy dosage on Monday. I have no sore mouth, no sore gums, no sores on my lips or in my mouth, no sore scalp and no flushing! Not even any headaches or nausea from the added IV iron treatment. Of course I do have the expected hyper task mode side effect of the Prednisone, but that is very manageable and temporary.

What happened? What changed? Dr. Patel told me the effects of chemotherapy drugs on the body were cumulative, so it stands to reason I would have had more side effects from this treatment, but I haven't so far. And with all the other treatments, whatever side effects I was going to have, I had within the first two or three days following treatment. And today is my third day since treatment and nothing has happened yet.

Could the miracle I had while in my chemotherapy treatment on Monday be the reason? Did I release some hidden resentment toward my treatment I didn't realize I had? I know when I was struggling trying to get Millie to leave I was feeling a bit like Jacob from the *Holy Bible*. Jacob struggled mightily with his troubles until he reached a point of being able to bless them. Once he could bless them, they released him and were gone ... forever.

So did I have such an experience during my meditation when I, at last, could bless the cancer rather than be angry at it and recognize "Millie" for his contribution to my healing? It was at that point that the angel appeared to collect "Millie" and I heard the message "your cancer is all gone" and then I felt the whoosh of release throughout my body.

There is no way to definitively know, but I know. It is over. I have learned the lessons I need to learn from this experience of cancer, and I'm grateful for the experience at last. I think it's impossible to have a cancer diagnosis and not have it be a life changing experience. For me it's a good change, and indeed I'm truly grateful.

I decide to write another affirmation confirming my commitment to listen and care for myself and my body:

I listen to myself

and my body;

I love myself

and I honor myself;

I love my body and

take care of my body;

My body is my true partner in life.

We are a great team!

Thank you!

As I began to write this morning, I had one of those moments ... an aha moment. Ever since I was diagnosed with cancer in July, I have written a "Daily Cancer Journal (date)" and this heading has been in my computer on every day, every month since then ... until today.

As I typed in the heading for today's journal, I was jolted by what I was writing. I knew I needed to change it for today and every day going forward. My title now is "Daily Healing Journal (date)". What a difference to change that one word. From cancer journal to healing journal. Profound actually. Hopefully it is another sign that my cancer is all gone and I am healed.

Now that it has been nearly two weeks since my fifth and next to last chemotherapy treatment, I still have had no side effects. Based on my experiences with previous treatments, I won't have any side effects in this last week either. Even when I had the more severe side effects after the first treatment, by the time I reached the third week, all side effects were resolved and nothing else emerged.

I'm thinking there must be some connection to my ability to relax during chemotherapy infusion and my level of side effects. For the first three treatments I was most scared, had elevated blood pressure beforehand the day of treatment and had the most difficulty relaxing into the treatment. And it was after these treatments that I experienced the side effects.

For the third treatment I had added music to help me relax, and it was after this infusion that I had the least side effects out of the first three. However, for treatment numbers four and five, I had normal blood pressure beforehand, and used a sleep mask and music to help me relax during the infusion. In fact meditation and music lulled me to sleep and I slept during a good part of the infusion.

While I have no scientific evidence this could be so, I do think there must be a connection between the state of my mind during infusion, the relaxed state of my body and the ability of my body to accept and process the chemicals coming into it. I am witnessing this very change.

Chapter 23

Closing in on the Finish

One last chemotherapy treatment. It seems hard to believe they are coming to a close. Everything has been built around healing this cancer for the past few months. Who knew a lump under my left lower eyelid could be so complicated to diagnose and heal?

It took three doctors and a biopsy before identifying the lump as cancer. And then once I knew it was cancer, some options for treatment were closed to me. First, surgical removal wasn't possible. Dr. Gallo, the eye and facial plastic surgeon performing the biopsy, was planning to remove it, but couldn't because of the cancer's location. The lump had grown under my eye and intertwined in the eye muscle. Not possible to remove without damage to my eye muscle, or perhaps my eye even.

And then radiation was also not likely as a treatment option. Again the location of the cancer made it a difficult cancer to treat with radiation without risk to damaging or losing my eyesight. A risk I was unwilling to take.

Well, I couldn't just leave the cancer in there, could I? That option would surely cause the loss of my eyesight as my eye would become more and more tilted upward due to the growth of the cancer. And the longer the cancer remained in my body, the more likely rogue cells could break away and set up housekeeping somewhere else in my body.

With surgery and radiation removed as options to treat my incurable lymphoma cancer that left chemotherapy as the only practical option. Definitely not my first choice, but once the decision was made, everything moved quickly

This process has been intense. I have learned so much about my body and the experience has deepened my love for it and my connection to it. I continue to eat a healthy diet every day with plenty of fresh fruits and vegetables. I think once the chemicals have finally left my body after the last chemotherapy treatment, my body will be completely clean on the inside and outside and I plan to do everything I can to keep it that way.

The change in my consciousness and awareness about my body is a miracle. Prior to the warning stroke I had 15 months ago, I never gave a thought to what I put into my body, nor what went on inside it. But after the stroke, I made a promise to love and take care of my body by eating healthily and less. That life style change is helping me to grow healthier and stronger every day.

My philosophy that it is never too late to change, grow or get an education is definitely working. Who knew a 74 year old could make such drastic changes in personal eating and exercise habits and become her own health and fitness advocate? I am living proof it is possible to have success at any age. I am witnessing tangible improvements in my health and now no longer need blood pressure medication.

Moving my body daily has resulted in being able to walk at least a mile every day, when beforehand I could not walk to the corner without pain forcing me back.

I am beginning to live the affirmation I wrote more than a year ago. *"I am in excellent health with a very fit, strong and flexible body."* Visualizations and affirmations truly work to bring about change.

Walking every day has helped me grow stronger and I need that strength today. It is only 22 degrees out with a light dusting of snow on the sidewalks. Buddy and I are all bundled up to be out in this cold weather. I haven't missed a day walking during chemotherapy treatment, and I don't want to miss one now. Actually it is easier walking now that the ice on the sidewalk has melted, and Buddy is so happy to be on his walk that even he doesn't seem to mind the cold. Normally we pass other people out walking with their dogs ... but not this morning!

My children are amazed at me and my response to the cancer diagnosis that I received months ago. They were scared, possibly more scared for me than they ever have been, and of course they had no idea what to expect. But they all wanted to help me get through chemotherapy treatment in whatever way they could.

My daughter Rebecca offered to come from DC/MD to be with me after every chemo treatment thinking I would need a lot of help for the first few days after treatment. But she had just taken a new job and I asked her to wait until we could see what my response might be first before she made such serious plans. It turned out she didn't need to make this sacrifice after all. I have been able to remain self sufficient throughout my entire chemotherapy treatment.

My daughter Suzanne, who lives only six miles from me, also felt drawn to be available and help me in any way I might need. She had just signed up to take two college classes when she learned I was to go through chemotherapy. Her first thought was to cancel both of them. I literally begged her not to delay her plans and cancel them. I'm grateful she finally listened to me as this sacrifice wasn't needed for her to be able to help me. Suzanne has driven me to every chemotherapy treatment and stayed the entire day, which is exactly how I did need help. It worked out perfectly that my chemotherapy was always scheduled on a Monday and her classes were on Tuesday and Thursday.

My son John did make a sacrifice for me by moving in with his girlfriend, giving me my best option to stay infection free. He was very worried for me saying he had firsthand knowledge of people going through chemotherapy and their reactions. While he was working, he transported patients to medical appointments. Many were senior passengers going through chemotherapy. He said most just gave up and collapsed not being able to do anything to help themselves.

I promised John I would not give up. I promised John I would do everything I could possibly do to take care of myself. I don't know if he really felt reassured at the time, but he knows I have kept my word. He is quite surprised at how well I have managed during treatment. He offered to do my grocery shopping for me, but fortunately I have been able to do my own shopping. I just wear a mask and gloves to protect myself.

I am grateful to my children for their loving support. I have felt loved, cared for and cared about every minute. One day my friend Jeannetta called to check on me and she shared she was worried I might be bored or lonely since I had decided not to attend any groups during treatment. I was pleased to reassure her that I was neither bored nor lonely at all. With daily phone calls from my children, writing every day and taking care of myself, my days are very rewarding and busy.

And I am very happy that I continue to learn new ways to take care of myself. Throughout chemotherapy, I have done everything I know to take care of myself. I have eaten nutritious food, kept myself hydrated, exercised every day, prepared food in advance, sanitized everything before a treatment, used meditations, prayer, visualizations and affirmations to help my healing. And I have written every day expressing gratitude for my life and the healing taking place. With all things working together, I have remained in good spirits with a very positive attitude.

To say my children are proud of me is an understatement. And in the process I have inspired them to be more aware and kindly toward their bodies. I am most proud of that. Who knew that this experience would bring us all even closer together?

My daughter Suzanne has witnessed my progress first hand on a daily basis. Although I haven't done it all perfectly and had some down days, she marvels how my unwavering faith has sustained me throughout ever since my cancer diagnosis. Just knowing in my heart of hearts that whatever happens will be for my highest good, leads me through whatever challenge I face. And it has inspired me to see her own faith grow as we have gone through this experience together.

This unwavering faith of mine is something that was created over a lifetime, and it definitely wasn't a linear experience. Until I was 13 years of age I had never been inside a church. That year I finally did attend one, and I went alone. While walking to school one day I saw an invitational sign for a revival at the Sydenstricker Methodist Church, located not far from where I lived at the time. I felt drawn to be there.

That evening service was one of those life changing moments for me. I responded to the call to be saved while listening to the song *Just As I Am*. All my deepest and hidden longings for love and acceptance came rushing forth and I couldn't hold back my emotions. It seemed impossible that someone, or something, could really want me and accept me just as I am. But I felt it. It must be true. While sobbing, a gentle force literally lifted me out of my seat, and without ever feeling my feet on the floor, I literally floated to the front of the church. Jesus entered my open heart at that moment, and his presence has been with me ever since.

Everyone came up to me afterwards, smiling, happy and inviting me to participate in their church. This was a new experience for me and I was thrilled to have people talk to me and want to include me. They even invited me to attend their Youth Fellowship meetings on Sunday evenings. I did attend the next Sunday evening meeting, and while there I met Jack Rosebrough. This was his mother's church. Little did I realize how much this coincidental meeting would change my life forever.

I continued attending this Methodist church on my own until I moved in with my sister and her family a few months later. My brother-in-law's family was heavily invested in the Baptist Church and he insisted I attend their church with them. I did, until I no longer lived with them, and then I tried other churches. I participated in the Episcopal, Presbyterian, Catholic, and Orthodox churches and I studied with a Buddhist Priest, a Swami and a Shaman.

I was always looking for the place where I belonged, where things made sense to me. But I never found the perfect fit. Something from each helped me, taught me more about God, the universe and deepened my faith. For years seeking, I now feel blessed with a wonderfully direct connection with God ... talking with him through my writing and prayer and listening to him through meditation ... and finally I have the connection and belonging that I searched for my whole life.

This lifetime of a puzzle has come together for me in a solid spiritual life where I live in love, joy, kindness, compassion, forgiveness and understanding. And best of all is my unwavering faith that everything works out for the best in the end ... no matter how it appears at the moment. Matthew 19:26 from the *Holy Bible* captures it best ... *with God all things are possible.*

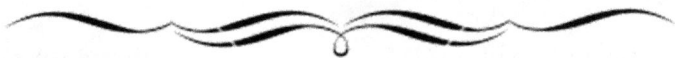

I believe my faith will

sustain me

whatever the challenge.

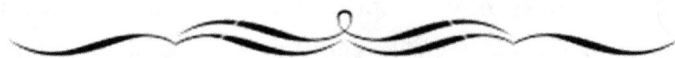

Chapter 24

Living My New Normal

Today is my last regularly scheduled chemotherapy treatment in the plan developed by Dr. Patel last August. As usual I did everything possible to be ready in advance. I sanitized the bathrooms, washed and changed my bed linens, the mattress cover and comforter, and I prepared my food and drinks for the day. I also packed my sleep mask, my CD player and meditative CDs, my gloves and my blanket.

My appointment is at 10:15 AM, two hours later than usual, so I even have a chance to walk my dog Buddy in the daylight before leaving. And my daughter and I totally miss the morning rush hour traffic getting onto the highway. With no traffic we make it to the appointment early. It's a good start to the day for sure.

While waiting for my appointment, Suzanne and I come up with a list of questions for Dr. Patel. Shortly after we meet for our appointment, he asks what is happening with me, if I have anything new to report and if I had side effects from the last treatment. I respond that I had no side effects from the last two treatments, except for the hyper activity from the Prednisone. I also tell him I have a list of questions for him and ask when I can ask those. He tells me to go ahead and begin my questions right then.

167

"I have been curious, Dr. Patel, if my particular type of cancer is slow growing and chemo drugs work to kill fast growing cancer cells, how will they work for me?"

Dr. Patel smiles and responds, "I wondered when you would ask that question." And then he moves closer to me on his roller chair with his yellow legal pad. He begins by drawing a diagram to explain how it will work for me. "As you can see from this line, you can imagine a car on the highway ... this first one might be going 75 miles an hour ... fast ... and the second one might be going only 60 or 65 miles an hour, fast, right, but not as fast as the first one. And over here at the beginning of the line, closer to zero, is the regular cell growth. So even though your cancer cells are considered slow growing because they are low level, they are still fast growing in comparison to regular cell activity. And that is how the chemotherapy will help you."

"Okay, next question ... did my iron IV infusion at the last treatment help to improve my anemia? And are the low red blood cells and hemoglobin the specific blood types that alerted you I am anemic?"

"No, there hasn't been any positive change there yet. In fact both are still low and may not come back completely until you are no longer receiving the chemo drugs. And yes, these are the two low counts that alerted me."

Then my daughter Suzanne asked him, "Should she be taking an iron supplement at home to help?"

"No, this IV iron she is receiving during one treatment is the equivalent of receiving one month of an iron supplement taken at home."

I speak up then and ask, "What about the immature grans #? If that is not zero is that an indication I still have some cancer cells?"

"No, it's only a matter of the timing of the test and what is happening in your body when it is taken. Cancer cells are dying all the time and a test at any given point in time might have a different result."

There's more that I want to know about what my options are so I ask Dr. Patel, "In my original diagnosis you said there could be six to eight chemotherapy treatments and I have had only six in this first plan. If the cancer is not all gone when I have the next PET body scan, is it likely I could continue with these two additional chemo treatments? And if I have just a sliver remaining under my eye, is it likely that surgery might be an option to remove it at that stage?"

As usual Dr. Patel is patient, kind and extremely helpful with his answers. He explains that this lymphoma is considered a liquid cancer and surgery is not a solution for it. Unfortunately I didn't ask him to define what liquid meant, but I can imagine.

Again he begins with his yellow pad drawing a diagram to illustrate my options. "If the cancer cells are all gone, or if there is no change in the results from your next PET scan, you will go to a maintenance mode of treatment. If you have no change, that means the chemotherapy is no longer working and it would not be helpful to continue. Of course if the cancer cells are all gone, there is no need for further chemotherapy treatment."

That was one direction on his diagram. Then he explains the alternative option. "If, however, there is improvement showing in the results, but there are some cancer cells remaining, you will have the extra two chemotherapy treatments we discussed in the beginning of your treatment."

Off to the side he also puts down radiation as an option for me if I am interested. When he shows me that I ask him, "Well, what about potential eyesight damage from this option?"

He replies, "This is an option if you are interested, but there is no guarantee that you would not have eyesight damage."

"Well, no thanks, as long as there is another option, I would rather not even consider radiation."

I'm still reeling from hearing the news about needing to go to a maintenance mode of treatment. I assumed that when the cancer was all gone I would just walk away and have periodic scans checking for any new cancer cell growth. Wrong. The diagram continues.

Dr Patel gives me a moment for it all to sink in and then goes on, "When you move into the maintenance mode, you won't need the chemo drugs. You will only receive the Rituximab. However, if you would stop treatment now, the research reports that this cancer could return in as little as 18 months. By going into maintenance mode, with treatments every other month for the next two years, we can delay the cancer's return up to 40 months or longer."

My goodness sakes. I will be in treatment for two more years and have to be on watch for the cancer's return for the rest of my life!! I guess that's what Dr. Patel told me on my very first treatment, that this particular cancer is very treatable, but not curable. Now I know for sure what that means to me. *I have incurable cancer!* I think I have been in denial of this fact. Somehow hearing the words this cancer is very treatable, but not curable, doesn't sound quite as serious to me as *I have incurable cancer!*

However, there is good news and bad news regarding transitioning to a maintenance mode and what I will be receiving. The bad news is that the maintenance mode includes treatments every other month for the next two years. The good news is I will only receive the Rituximab drug during maintenance mode, and neither of the chemo drugs I have been receiving during this initial chemotherapy treatment. This means I should be able to avoid the side effects that I have had so far ... as they were all from the chemo drugs.

And after going through all these initial treatments, the speed of my being able to absorb the Rituximab has improved from the lengthy 4 hours in my first treatment to only 90 minutes. That will be the fastest absorption rate I can expect during maintenance mode. I will continue to receive the Benedryl along with the Rituximab since it curbs side effects. But Benedryl usually makes me very drowsy so I may still need someone to drive me to these treatments.

Before I got all this information about shifting into a maintenance mode, even if the cancer is all gone now, I asked Dr. Patel, "when do you think I can plan to have my port removed?"

That question opened the door to the whole conversation about maintenance mode, but his response to my question was ... "You'll be wearing it all your life ... "

Now that was a sobering thought and actually prepared me to hear why I would be needing it.

I regretted not following up with a question to Dr. Patel to explain what the term liquid cancer meant, so I checked the Internet when I got home to see what I could find out. It was easy. Immediately I found great information from the University of Michigan Comprehensive Cancer Center on their uofmhealthblogs.org website.

They refer to leukemia and lymphomas as "liquid tumors". Also called blood cancers, these cancers affect the bone marrow, the blood cells and the lymphatic system. Every 4 minutes, 1 person in the United States is diagnosed with a blood cancer according to the Leukemia and Lymphoma Society. Leukemia and lymphoma are often grouped together and considered related cancers because they probably all result from acquired mutations to the DNA of a single lymph-or blood-forming stem cell.

And they list the number one common treatment as chemotherapy. They also list the chemo drugs that I am currently receiving as the drugs of choice for treatment.

This news stuns me. My mother died of leukemia! I never once gave a thought that my having an incurable lymphoma cancer now could have any connection to my family acquired genetics. But of course it does!

My mother, who was 42 at the time I was born, was quite ill while she was pregnant with me. Sometime around the time I was born she had all her teeth pulled and suffered severe bleeding. She continued to be on bed rest for some time. My older sister, only 14 at the time, was my major caregiver that first summer of my life. Unfortunately she also had all the other household responsibilities of cooking, laundry, cleanup, and watching out for my two older brothers. No wonder I have had this recurring vision of being on the dining room table as an infant, no clothes on, arms and legs flailing and screaming my head off. My sister must have been changing my diaper and got called away for a bigger emergency.

Learning of my possible genetic link to my mother's illness makes me extremely grateful to Dr. Sparling, Dr. Calloway and Dr. Gallo. All of these doctors took me seriously until this cancer was identified while it was still in just one location in my body. Given that I had no other health issues to bring this cancer forth to be discovered, it could have remained in my body growing indefinitely, and sooner or later, possibly splitting off to other locations in my body.

With the changes I made in my lifestyle after having the warning stroke and receiving the diagnosis of incurable cancer, I have already created my new normal, and I will be living this new lifestyle the rest of my life.

Actually there is other good news about being on maintenance mode for the next two years. First, there could be a wonderful discovery in cancer research to help me prevent this cancer from ever returning. And then, since I am still pretty new taking care of myself and eating nutritious food, being on maintenance mode for that length of time will help keep me totally focused until my routine and choices become really solid.

If I do my part eating a healthy mostly plant based diet and exercise daily, I'm convinced that the cancer will never return. I will keep my dream boards posted, I will keep my affirmations posted, I will visualize being healthy, strong and fit, I will meditate that I am cancer free and I will value every minute of my life living as deliberately as I possibly can. I think the best is yet to come for me.

And I have had a glimpse of that new life coming forth. I emailed an unedited, unfinished draft manuscript to Zangmeister to review, prior to gaining their approval to use their name, and my doctor's name, in this book. They had no idea how much courage it took to share this manuscript which contains the shame and secrets of my past ... information that few people have ever heard about before.

Although I prepared myself for hearing "no," which would mean writing a generic version, I was more than delighted when I heard instead a resounding "Yes!" from the administration at Zangmeister. I could include their name and the doctors were excited about the book!! My secrets were out, and I wasn't shamed for sharing them!

All the other doctors had no idea what I might say in the book about them, but each and every one of them didn't hesitate to give me their wholehearted support and approval to be included. Hearing their enthusiasm was absolutely inspiring to me.

Crossing this hurdle means I have faced going public with my shame and more than survived, I thrived. The fear of going public in the past kept me from finishing and publishing my autobiography *Coal Dust to Diamonds*. Now I can do that with an open heart.

And if this book inspires just one person to improve their health and life by loving their body and taking care of it, then the joy I experienced writing this book will remain alive within me forever.

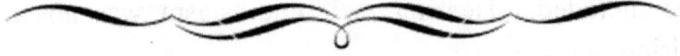

Love and be kind

to your

body.

It is your partner for life!

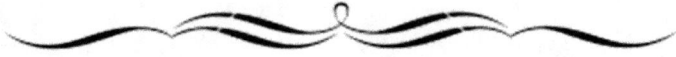

Epilogue

Today I received the results of my last PET body scan, and Dr. Patel told me what I already knew in my heart ... my cancer is all gone!! No more chemo! Now I move directly into maintenance mode. I was so deliriously happy when Dr. Patel gave me the news, I even yelled and did a tap dance while sitting in my chair.

Hearing officially that my cancer is gone is not only wonderful news, it is confirmation that I can trust whatever I receive in meditation. I feel validated that the vision about "Millie" and the "Your cancer is all gone" message I received were real, not just wishful thinking on my part.

I like rereading the PET scan results that Dr. Patel gave me ... "There has been *complete resolution* of asymmetrically prominent FDG localization about the left inferior rectus orbital muscle ... ".

All my family was with me for Christmas this year. We celebrated the end of my chemotherapy treatment and my success getting through it. Although we didn't have the results yet, all of us expressed gratitude for the cancer being gone. It is inspiring now to find out it really is gone. I feel truly blessed.

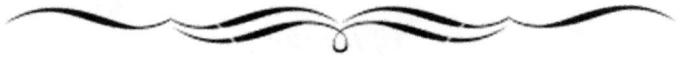

I have learned that when a red flag appears in a situation I am to take a different path. When I ignore the warning, I always encounter far greater pain.

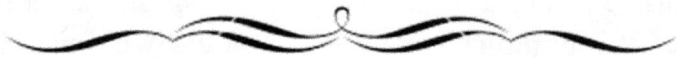

Exhibit I

Top Ten Healing Tools

1) Accept, appreciate, love and take care of your body

2) Eat Nutritiously and take healthy food with you on treatment days and when away from home

3) Hydrate consistently and take containers of water or your favorite healthy drink with you when you are away from home

4) Exercise daily

5) Prevent Infections/wash hands/sanitize

6) Meditate/Pray

7) Listen to meditative/uplifting music

8) Write about your healing journey

9) Visualize and write/post affirmations

10) Forgive ... yourself and others

Bonus Tip

Express gratitude daily for your healing and your life

Exhibit II

Solutions for My Side Effects

According to Dr. Nixon, my dermatologist, the skin is the largest organ in my body. This was new information to me as I had never considered the skin as an organ. Even more importantly, she shared that chemotherapy is a risk factor for melanoma skin cancer!

These facts become critical in chemotherapy as the drugs play havoc with the skin, especially inside the mouth and the scalp. It has a drying effect on the skin, can cause sores, make nails brittle, make the scalp sore or tender and many lose all their hair during treatment.

These things happen because chemotherapy drugs are designed to kill fast growing cancer cells. Unfortunately, at the same time they also attack healthy fast growing cells in the body which are in the mouth and hair follicles. Nearly all my side effects to chemo drugs occurred in these areas.

Solutions

For most solutions listed below I include the brand name product I selected to help me resolve the side effect.

Dry Skin

Dove liquid soap for sensitive skin for my showers.

Ivory, clean and simple liquid hand soap for hand soap dispensers.

Palmolive Soft Touch with Aloe for dry skin as dishwashing liquid detergent.

Fragrance free Curel body lotion. I use daily, immediately after my shower, all over my body to keep my skin moist. Fragrance free products help to curb my nausea sensitivity to aromas.

Clear ... for Scalp and Hair shampoo and conditioner, very nourishing for my tender scalp and non irritating; and prescriptions Betamethasone Dipropionate and Taclonex.

Curel's *Rough Skin Rescue* for dry and cracking skin on my hands due to excessive washing. I also alternate using coconut oil and cocoa butter; these are also very helpful.

Aquaphor lip balm to repair my dry and cracking lips.

Abreva to heal my lip sores.

Lukewarm water instead of very hot for my showers; it is less drying for the skin.

Fragrance free laundry detergent.

Sore Mouth & Gums

"Magic Mouthwash" prescription. Before that was available I had to stop flossing and switch from electric toothbrushes to soft bristle toothbrushes. With it my mouth and gums healed enough to resume flossing and using electric toothbrushes.

Flushing

Benedryl relieved the redness and burning heat in my face from flushing. When Benedryl didn't work I was advised to stop taking the Prednisone prescription.

Nausea

Anti-nausea prescription medication and switching to fragrance free products when possible.

Constipation

Stool softeners.

Hyper Task Mode

Once I knew that Prednisone did not elevate my blood pressure or temperature, and that my only reaction was the hyper task mode, I made it work for me. I used the extra energy to write this book ... while going through chemotherapy treatment!

Exhibit III

Steps to Prevent Infection

Following are the steps I used daily to prevent infections during chemotherapy and I will continue to use these steps daily to help keep myself healthy.

Wash hands ... consistently and frequently

Use paper towels to dry hands and recycle/discard.

Use a plastic spoon for coconut oil or cocoa butter and recycle, discard or wash before reusing.

Wash all fruits and vegetables before eating or cutting.

Don't share bath towels and wash cloths. Change daily.

Keep mouth clean with frequent flossing, brushing and mouth wash.

Keep sanitizing wipes in bathrooms to wipe down toilet seats and handles.

Use sanitizing wipes to clean light switches, door handles, cabinet handles, computer keys, remotes, especially before treatment.

Change bed linens regularly, especially before a treatment.

Use face mask and gloves when dusting and vacuuming. (I have even been using a face mask and gloves for grocery shopping.)

Limit activity in crowds.

Exhibit IV

My Blood Test Results Vs. Normal Ranges

	Results Pre Chemo	*Normal Ranges*	*Post Chemo*
WBC	7.13	4.4 - 11.0	6.48
RBC	4.34	4.1 - 5.43	3.73
HGB	13.3	11.9 - 16.0	11.3
HCT	39.6	36.0 - 47.0	34.7
MCV	91.2	80.0 - 99.0	93.0
MCH	30.6	27.0 - 31.7	30.3
MCHC	33.6	32.3 - 36.0	32.6
RDW	12.5	11.6 - 16.5	13.8
Platelet Count	235	140 - 449.0	201
Granulocytes	3.8146	1.8 - 7.7	3.9334
Lymphocytes	2.5312	1.0 - 4.8	1.6718
Monocytes	0.4991	0.1 - 0.9	0.6998
Eosinophils	0.1497	0.0 - 0.45	0.1231
Basophils	0.1283	0.0 - 0.2	0.0518
MPV	8.9	7.4 - 11.0	8.1
Immat Grans #	0.01	0.0 - 0.0	0.00

Source: The Mark H. Zangmeister Center/my medical reports

References

Books

The Holy Bible, Authorized King James Version, Thomas Nelson Bibles, 2003 by Thomas Nelson, Inc., Matthew 6:9-13 *The Lord's Prayer;* Genesis 32:24-26, Jacob and blessing; Matthew 19:26 *With God all things are possible.*

Holliman, Jeannetta, *Works in Process: Women Over 50 Reflecting,* 2014, Biblio Publishing, Columbus, Ohio

Saraswati, Swami Shantanand "Shantji" - *Are You Free? The Mystical Wisdom of "Non Doing"* Shanti Temple, Montrose PA 18801, *2001 pp 18-22 (description of Non-Doing).*

Whitfield, Charles L., M.D. *Healing the Child Within,* Health Communications, Inc., Deerfield Beach FL, 1987 pp 52 -53 *(description of age regression)*

Funeral Home/Cemeteries/Vault Company

Flint Cemetery, 8187 Flint Road, Worthington, Ohio 43085

Phillips Funeral Home, 1004 S. 7th Street, Ironton, Ohio 45638

Tri-State Wilbert Vault, PO Box 231, Ironton Ohio 45638

Woodland Cemetery, 824 Lorain Street, Ironton, Ohio 45638

Education

Betsy Magness Leadership Institute (BMLI), Women in Cable Telecommunications, 2000 K Street, N.W. Suite 350, Washington DC, www.wict.org

Coach University, a global leader in coach training, www.coachu.com.

Franklin University, 201 South Grant Street, Columbus OH 43215, an accredited non-profit college offering bachelor and master degree programs, www.franklin.edu.

Retirement Options, a retirement coach training/certification program; 6390 Quadrangle Drive, Ste. 160, Chapel Hill NC 27517, www.retirementoptions.com.

Medical

Jason Barfield, M.D., Mount Carmel Neurology, St Ann's, 495 Cooper Road Suite 211, Westerville Oh 43081

George F. Calloway, Jr., M.D., Central Ohio Ophthalmology, Inc., St. Ann's Medical Office Bldg., 495 Cooper Road, Westerville OH 43081

Mark E. Davanzo, M.D., General Surgery, 477 Cooper Road, Suite 440, Westerville OH 43081

Samuel A. Gallo, M.D., Gallo Eye and Facial Plastic Surgery, 6620 Perimeter Dr., Ste. 100 Dublin, OH 43016

Leukemia & Lymphoma Society, 1311 Mamaroneck Avenue, Suite 310, White Plains NY 10605, www.lls.org

Loving Yourself Through Cancer

Liquid tumor description - www.uofmhealthblogs.org

Ramona M. Sarsama Nixon, D.O., Board Certified
Dermatologist, 44 S Kintner Parkway, Suite B, Sunbury OH
43074

Omron, www.omron-healthcare.com (blood pressure
monitoring equipment)

Taral Patel, M.D., my oncology specialist, The Mark H.
Zangmeister Center, 3100 Plaza Properties Blvd., Columbus
OH 43219.

Monica Pesa, Director of Nursing, Perimeter Surgical
Center, 6620 Perimeter Dr. Ste. 100, Dublin OH 43016

PET scan, Positron Emission Tomography, reveals presence
and severity of cancers. www.petscaninfo.com

Wendy L. Sparling, D.O., Sunbury Square Family Medicine,
27 N Vernon Street, Sunbury OH 43074

Brittany Sweigart, CNP, The Mark H. Zangmeister Center,
3100 Plaza Properties Blvd., Columbus OH 43219

The Mark H. Zangmeister Center, *The Choice for Oncology
& Hematology,* 3100 Plaza Properties Blvd. Columbus OH
43219. www.zangcenter.com

Music

Bernhardt, Patrick *Atlantis Angelis,* Shining Star Music,
Atlantis Angelis Network, 1600 de Lorimier, Montreal,
Canada H2K 3W5, 2002

Elliott, Charlotte, composer of *Just As I* Am, 1835

Hammerstein, Oscar II (lyrics) and Rogers, Richards (music) *I'm Gonna Wash That Man Right Outa My Hair* from 1949 Broadway Musical *South Pacific.* Sheet music owned by Williamson Music.

Wai Lana & Siddha *Yoga Sound*, Gold Moon Productions, PO Box 146, Malibu CA 90264, 1998

Nutrition Websites

Please note that the information on all the following websites is available at no charge and no subscription is required.

www.caloriecount.about.com - Easy way to get nutrient ingredients and calories of individual foods.

www.cnpp.usda.gov - Center for Nutrition Policy and Promotion

www.fitnessmagazine.com - healthy eating recipes and fitness tips; a free email service is also available for recipes and fitness suggestions.

www.Theppk.com - my daughter Rebecca's favorite vegan website with a tremendous selection of vegan recipes. It also has a blog for interaction.

www.usda.gov; I found the dietary guidelines extremely helpful as I navigated to healthy eating every day.

Sacred and Cleansing Rituals

Sage - an ancient and sacred herb used in smudging ceremonies by Native Americans for thousands of years to cleanse, bless, and protect a person or space. I use it when I want to clear away negativity or bless an area, such as a new home. I light the edge of the sage stick until smoke easily emerges. If there is an active flame, I blow that out. Smudging is using the smoke to cleanse or bless an area while saying a prayer. www.shamansmarket.com; www.taosherbs.com/sage

Incense - The rising smoke of incense has come to symbolize prayers rising up to God. In The Old Testament of the *Holy Bible,* Psalm 141:2, there is a plea ... "Let my prayer be set forth before thee as incense ..." www.biblemeanings.info/Words/Plant/Incense

Safety

www.32north.com - website for Stable Icers ice cleats

Writing Group

International Women's Writing Guild, New York NY, www.iwwg.org

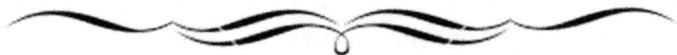

I am filled with gratitude.

My cancer is

totally and completely gone

Now and forevermore!

Thank you!

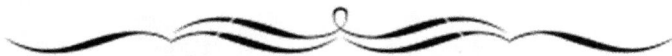

About the Author

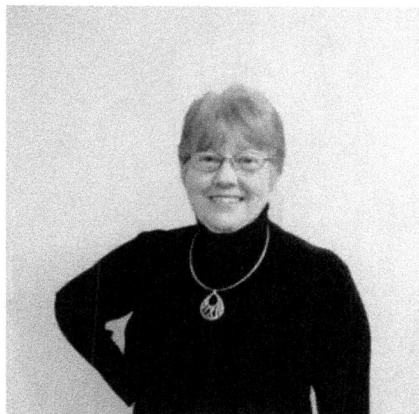

Carol Rosebrough is a retired executive from the cable television industry where she received many accolades, including being selected as one of *Pennsylvania's Best 50 Women in Business.* She graduated from Franklin University in Columbus, Ohio with a degree in Business Administration, Coach University as a Life Coach and received certification as a Retirement Coach through Retirement Options.

Since retirement, Carol now enjoys her time with family and writing. She was most recently published as a contributing author in the anthology *Works in Process: Women Over 50 Reflecting.*

At the age of 74 she added cancer survivor to her list of accomplishments. This book is the story of her journey, lessons learned, and the tools she used to help herself heal and remain positive throughout treatment. Carol believes the answers to one's life are found by looking within and that it is never too late to learn, change and grow. *Loving Yourself Through Cancer,* written as she was going through chemotherapy, provides hope and inspiration that healing can be achieved at any age.

www.crosebrough.com

lovingyourself@crosebrough.com